NATURAL BEAUTY SECRETS FROM INDIA

NATURAL BEAUTY SECRETS FROM INDIA

EASY, ECONOMICAL, *AND* EFFECTIVE
HEAD-TO-TOE HOME REMEDIES
FOR A BEAUTIFUL YOU, NATURALLY

Roshni Dayal

TATE PUBLISHING & *Enterprises*

Natural Beauty Secrets from India
Copyright © 2008 by Roshni Dayal. All rights reserved.

This title is also available as a Tate Out Loud product. Visit www.tatepublishing.com for more information.

No part of this publication may be reproduced, stored in a retrieval system or transmitted in any way by any means, electronic, mechanical, photocopy, recording or otherwise without the prior permission of the author except as provided by USA copyright law.

The opinions expressed by the author are not necessarily those of Tate Publishing, LLC.

Published by Tate Publishing & Enterprises, LLC
127 E. Trade Center Terrace | Mustang, Oklahoma 73064 USA
1.888.361.9473 | www.tatepublishing.com

Tate Publishing is committed to excellence in the publishing industry. The company reflects the philosophy established by the founders, based on Psalm 68:11,
"The Lord gave the word and great was the company of those who published it."

Book design copyright © 2008 by Tate Publishing, LLC. All rights reserved.
Cover design by Roshni Dayal and Kellie Southerland
Interior design by Roshni Dayal and Stefanie Rooney

Published in the United States of America
ISBN: 978-1-60604-918-1
1. Health and Fitness: Beauty and Grooming: General
2. Health and Fitness: Alternative Therapies
08.08.27

PRAISE

"Skin care and premature aging are topics that most women are concerned about. We collectively spend billions of dollars each year on products that will enable us to look younger and healthier. In many cases, these products contain chemicals that are harmful to our skin.

Natural Beauty Secrets from India is filled with remedies using ingredients that are pure *and* inexpensive. I was experiencing a lot of trouble with dry skin. Upon Roshni's recommendation, I immediately started using a mixture of Olive and Vitamin E oils. I was amazed at how supple my skin became within just a few days—I can't wait to try more of these remedies!

This book is a 'must have' for *all* women!"

Janey Hays, Acquisitions Representative, Tate Publishing & Enterprises, LLC

"I suffered from severe acne for almost ten years. I tried everything on the market from Murad to Proactiv. Nothing seemed to work. Frustrated and confused, but still desperate to clear my skin, I decided to opt for laser treatment. However, Roshni urged me to try one of the home remedies in her book. Having learned not to hold any expectations whatsoever, I agreed to try the Honey and Cinnamon mask. In just three days, I saw a noticeable difference. I continued to use the mask for the remainder of three weeks. The results were astonishing—my beautiful skin had emerged!

Natural Beauty Secrets from India focuses on simple, yet effective, solutions for the most common problems that we all encounter. I *definitely* plan on recommending this book to all my clients!"

Janrace Prudent, Fashion and Beauty Consultant, Sparkle Eyes / www.sparkleyes.com

DISCLAIMER

This book is the result of extensive research and is designed to provide accurate and reliable information regarding the subject matter covered. The information provided herein is not a substitute for medical, health or professional advice. The information is further furnished with the understanding that neither the author nor the publisher is engaged in rendering medical, health or professional advice of any kind. Given that the details of your situation are fact dependent, you should seek the services of a licensed professional to discuss *any* circumstances that apply to you, before and during the use of these remedies. Also, read the SAFETY PRECAUTIONS in the section titled, "**READ ME FIRST!**" before you use *any* ingredient referenced herein.

Further, neither the author nor the publisher makes any warranty, express or implied, including the warranty of merchantability and fitness for a particular purpose, or assumes any legal liability or responsibility for any risk undertaken or damage incurred, directly or indirectly, as a result of *any* of the remedies contained herein, the variance of their results, or the accuracy, completeness, or usefulness of *any* information, apparatus, product, ingredient, remedy or process disclosed, or represents that its use would not infringe any privately owned rights.

Finally, reference herein to any specific commercial product, ingredient, remedy, process, service by trade name, trademark, manufacturer, or otherwise, does not necessarily constitute or imply its endorsement, recommendation, or favoring, and nor does it constitute or imply its disparagement by the author or the publisher.

DEDICATION

To My Beloved Parents,

I sit here, faced with an extremely difficult task of expressing in a few words, the gratitude I hold in my heart for being born to the both of you. Words can't do justice to the sacrifices that you made, so that I could turn out to be the human being you hoped I would be. Thank you for worrying about me *every* step of the way and for encouraging me to *always* see the silver lining in the clouds—it has allowed me to gracefully find my happiness every time I've had a disheartening day. Thank you for showing me how to be grateful for all things, big and small. And thank you for teaching me to be curious to learn—I remember, Dad, that you said to me, "If you ask a question, you may perhaps look ignorant for a minute, but if you *don't* ask it, you will look ignorant for a lifetime!"

Both of you raised me to be humble, yet strong. You instilled in me the very morals and principles that have allowed you to hold your heads high in your own journeys through life. You showed me how to smile from my heart. It is from you that I learned to appreciate the beauty in simplicity.

From the bottom of my heart, I dedicate my book to you with a strong awareness that if it weren't for your blessings, I wouldn't have made it this far. *You are, and always will be with me!*

Your Loving Daughter,

Roshni

TABLE OF CONTENTS

READ ME FIRST!	1
HAIR AND SCALP	5
Oily Hair	6
Dull or Dry Hair	8
Breakage and Split Ends	12
Premature Graying	13
Hair Loss	15
Dandruff	18
Shampoo and Styling Product Build-Up	21
EYES	23
Eyebrows and Eyelashes	24
Tired Eyes	25

Puffy Eyes	26
Dark Circles	28

FACE **31**

Oily Skin	35
Dry Skin	37
Dark or Dull Complexion	39
Uneven Pigmentation	42
Freckles	44
Clogged Pores and Blackheads	45
Pimples, Acne, and Blemishes	49
Premature Aging	55
Fine Lines and Wrinkles	58
Unwanted Facial Hair	61
Dry or Chapped Lips	63
Attain a Smooth and Radiant Complexion	64

NECK **67**

ARMS, TORSO, AND LEGS 69

NAILS 75

FEET 79

MAKE YOUR OWN BEAUTY ESSENTIALS 83
Cleansers, Astringents, and Toners 85
Natural Exfoliants 88
Facemasks 90

ABOUT THE INGREDIENTS 95

WHERE YOU CAN FIND THE INGREDIENTS 121

READ ME FIRST!

Day after day, a wasteful abundance of man-made beauty products continues to bury our store shelves. Their manufacturers spend billions of dollars on their marketing and advertising through *every* medium, in an effort to make us believe that we are not spending enough on ourselves. These over-the-counter products are proclaimed to be "new-age miracles"—they promise to eliminate the need for cosmetic surgery and various laser treatments. Most, however, do not deliver the extent of what they promise and have led a large number of people to opt for alternative, invasive forms of remedial treatment. In turn, over and above the physical and financial discomfort that accompany them, these alternative procedures are proving that they can *also* come with their fair share of side effects. This is, ultimately, now leading many to look for simpler and more economical ways to achieve the same aesthetic results.

In exploring our options, we steadily see more and more natural ingredients being incorporated into many beauty products on the market today—cucumbers, honey, milk, papaya, olive oil—to name just a few. Unfortunately, these ingredients form only a *fraction* of the product's content; yet, the creators of the product claim that it is close to nature—they package it in attractive

containers and slap on a premium price, now placing it in a category that meets all the requirements to generate appeal (*and, of course,* revenue).

So, if just *a meager* presence of natural ingredients contributes to the appeal of the product, then you will not disagree that using these very ingredients *directly* onto your hair and skin, without all the added chemicals, perfumes, and preservatives, can only benefit you. After all, most of these ingredients are a part of our diets, and if they are nutritious enough to keep us healthy on the inside, then they *must* be better alternatives to the chemically-induced beauty products that, if ingested, advise us on their labels to call the Poison Hotline—*Food for Thought!*

In addition to raising your awareness on the benefits of natural ingredients, my intention through this book is to let you know that *even if you can* afford expensive products, more money doesn't necessarily translate to better results—there's a lot you can do for yourself aesthetically, using natural home remedies. Making your own beauty concoctions will not only cost a fraction of what you pay for over-the-counter products, but also, you will enjoy a sense of purity and freshness, which commercial products can't possibly offer you. So take a step back in time—the solutions that you seek so desperately could be sitting in your *very own* kitchen!

READ ME FIRST!

NOTES

- ❀ This book is not about makeup application tricks. It will not teach you how to conceal your imperfections; instead, it will provide you with natural, effective, *and* inexpensive ways to reduce, or even cure, them. Although you may begin to see positive changes with your very first use of these remedies, desirable results do take time and dedication to achieve, so do not lose your patience.

- ❀ For your convenience, any remedy that forms the solution to more than one problem has been repeated in that problem's respective section. As you concoct your remedies, I strongly urge you to refer to the section, "**ABOUT THE INGREDIENTS**." You will read about the curative benefits of each ingredient and learn how it plays an important role in the remedy that you are employing.

SAFETY PRECAUTIONS

- ❀ Although many of the ingredients mentioned in this book are edible, all of the remedies contained herein are intended for external use only and are to be employed expressly for the purposes suggested.

- ❀ Do not use any ingredient referenced herein if you are aware of any sensitivity or allergy that you may have to that ingredient. Consult a licensed healthcare provider (and also test a small area of your skin well in advance) if you are unsure about using an ingredient. The responsibility to identify any adverse reaction and further exercise judgment regarding the use of each ingredient lies solely with the reader.

- ❀ These remedies are not a substitute for a faulty diet or lifestyle. We are what we put in our bodies and our personal choices affect not only our internal, but also our external health.

HAIR AND SCALP

Underneath its skin, our scalp harbors thousands of tiny sacs known as follicles, more commonly referred to as hair roots, in which our hair is formed. Our hair is made of a protein called keratin. A healthy scalp typically harbors approximately 100,000 strands of hair. Interestingly, every human being loses an average of sixty-to-eighty strands per day. This is very normal and doesn't quite constitute hair loss. Assuming that your scalp is not malnourished, your fallen strands will soon be replenished by newer, healthier ones, which will each grow between ¼ and ½ inch per month.

Lack of proper care for our hair and scalp, as well as the influence of several different factors—for example, an improper diet, hormonal imbalances, stress and anxiety, dry weather, or excessive exposure to the sun *or* salon procedures (including perming, coloring, and the use of heated styling appliances)—can all lead to unhealthy hair, dandruff, and even hair loss. While there are several home remedies to improve the quality of your hair, restore the nourishment to a dry scalp, and promote hair growth, over and above implementing these, also recognize the negative effects that the above factors can have on your hair and scalp, and make a conscious effort to limit your exposure to the ones that are within your control.

Oily Hair

- Add 3 tablespoons of lemon juice (*or* 3 tablespoons of apple cider vinegar) to 1 cup of warm water. After you shampoo, soak your hair with either mixture. Leave it on for approximately 5 minutes, and then rinse it off with tolerably cool water. (In the alternative, add 4–5 drops of lemon juice *or* 4–5 drops of apple cider vinegar directly to your dollop of shampoo—massage this mixture onto your hair and scalp, and then rinse it off as you normally would.) Both lemon juice and vinegar not only dissolve excess oil deposits on your scalp, but also effectively treat dandruff, infuse the shine back into your hair, and strip out any shampoo or styling product residue from your strands. (Note: While vinegar is known to add highlights to brunette hair, combined with heat, lemon juice also imparts highlights to hair. If you use the lemon juice mixture, let your hair dry naturally—do not sit out in the sun or use any heated appliances, such as a blow dryer.)

- If excess natural oils are weighing down your hair, add 1 raw egg to your dollop of shampoo. Wash your hair with this mixture to help it attain volume and bounce. (Note: Beware of rinsing your hair in hot water—the egg could scramble and become difficult to tease out!)

OILY HAIR

- In 1½ cups of water, boil 2 tablespoon's worth of fresh basil leaves (*or* 2 tablespoon's worth of fresh mint leaves) for 15–20 minutes. Strain the resulting liquid and store it in a bottle next to your shampoo; each time you wash your hair, mix the equivalent of 1 teaspoon of this solution with your dollop of shampoo.

- Conditioners are none other than moisturizers for our hair. If you have oily hair, then you already have more moisture than your hair normally needs; therefore, skip this step in your hair cleansing routine. (If the ends of your hair are dry, however, apply a small amount of conditioner directly onto them.)

- Brushing or combing our hair is, no doubt, an important step in our everyday grooming routine—it promotes healthy hair by increasing the circulation of blood to our scalp. The friction caused by the bristles or teeth, however, also activates the sebaceous (oil) glands in our scalp; the bristles or teeth themselves further distribute our natural oils from our scalp to our strands. Therefore, if you have oily hair, prevent the frequent transfer of oil from your scalp by brushing or combing your hair *no more than* once a day.

Dull or Dry Hair

- Oil conditions our hair wonderfully, coating and nourishing each strand and putting the sheen back into it. An oil massage also increases the blood circulation to our scalp, promoting hair growth. Gently massage some warm olive (*or* coconut *or* almond) oil onto your hair and scalp once a week, leaving it on for *at least* 1 hour before you shampoo. (Optional: Add 1 teaspoon of gooseberry powder to your oil—in addition to nourishing dull or dry hair, gooseberry also aids in curing premature graying, dandruff, and hair loss. If you choose to add this ingredient to your oil, leave the application on for *at least* 2 hours before you shampoo.)

- Oils like gooseberry and neem do wonders for our hair. Like any other oil, massage either of these gently onto your hair and scalp. Leave it on for *at least* 1 hour before you shampoo. These oils are very effective for not only infusing the sheen back into our hair, but also preventing or fighting dandruff *and* hair loss.

- Soak equal quantities of gooseberry and henna powders in just enough water to form a moderately thick paste. Instead of your usual shampoo, wash your hair with this mixture. Rinse with your regular conditioner. This remedy not only softens your hair and infuses the shine back

into it, but also promotes hair growth. (Note: Henna imparts a rich, brownish-red color to black or brunette hair. Its use also stains our skin, so make sure that you use a pair of gloves when you employ this remedy.)

- Add the white of 1 raw egg to your dollop of shampoo. Wash your hair with this mixture, and then rinse it until it is no longer slick. (Beware of rinsing your hair in hot water—the egg white could scramble and become difficult to tease out!)

- Add 3 tablespoons of lemon juice (*or* 3 tablespoons of apple cider vinegar) to 1 cup of warm water. After you shampoo, rinse your hair with either mixture. In addition to infusing the shine back into your hair, this remedy effectively treats oily hair and dandruff, as well as strips out any shampoo or styling product build-up from your strands. (Note: While vinegar is known to add highlights to brunette hair, combined with heat, lemon juice also imparts highlights to hair. If you use the lemon juice mixture, let your hair dry naturally—do not sit out in the sun or use any heated appliances, such as a blow dryer.)

- 20 minutes before you wash your hair, apply onto it a paste made from equal quantities of gram flour and plain yogurt. This remedy is also effective for treating breakage and split ends. (Note: Allow the yogurt

DULL OR DRY HAIR

to warm to room temperature before you apply this mixture—applying cold yogurt could cause a headache.)

- 20–30 minutes before you wash your hair, apply some glycerin onto it. If you have any oils at home—whether castor, almond, coconut, olive, gooseberry, *or* neem—mix any one in with the glycerin to reduce its thickness before you apply it.

- Mix some coconut cream powder in just enough water to form coconut milk that is creamy in consistency. Approximately 30 minutes before you shampoo, nourish your scalp and hair with this, making sure that you put on a shower cap to hold the coconut milk to your hair. (You can also use canned coconut milk; however, its shelf life is usually shorter than that of coconut cream powder. Furthermore, using the powdered form allows you to concoct just the quantity of coconut milk you need for this remedy, preventing any wastage.)

- Unless you oiled your hair, do not apply your shampoo more than once when you normally wash it—doing so robs your scalp and hair of your own natural oils.

- Hot water damages hair. When you wash your hair, make sure that you lower the temperature of your water, and in fact, before you turn off

DULL OR DRY HAIR

the shower, give your hair a tolerably cool rinse—this will seal your hair cuticles and lock in your natural oils.

- Brush or comb your hair daily—this increases the circulation of blood to the roots of your hair. Also, the friction caused by the bristles or teeth activates the sebaceous (oil) glands in your scalp; the bristles or teeth themselves further distribute your natural oils from your scalp to your strands, making your hair healthy and lustrous.

Breakage and Split Ends

- Blend to a smooth pulp 1 ripe banana and 1 tablespoon of almond oil. Apply this mixture onto your hair and leave it on for approximately 15 minutes before you shampoo.

- 20 minutes before you wash your hair, apply onto it a paste made from equal quantities of gram flour and plain yogurt. This remedy is also effective for treating dull or dry hair. (Note: Allow the yogurt to warm to room temperature before you apply this mixture—applying cold yogurt could cause a headache.)

- Use your conditioner moderately—over-conditioning can damage your hair and cause split ends. (If you do have split ends, prevent them from getting worse by scheduling a trim every four-to-six weeks.)

- Do not use rubber bands to tie your hair—they tend to break or split hair when they're taken off. Instead, use fabric-lined bands.

- Do not brush your hair when it's wet—it is the weakest and most elastic when wet and is likely to break off mid-strand. If you must detangle your hair, towel-dry it first and then *gently* detangle it using a wide-tooth comb. Even better, detangle it before you wash it, so that you can let it dry naturally.

Premature Graying

- Gooseberry makes an excellent remedy in slowing down the process of premature graying. It also helps cure other hair and scalp-related problems, such as dull or dry hair, dandruff, and hair loss. Mix 1 teaspoon of gooseberry powder with some warm olive, coconut, *or* almond oil and apply this paste onto your scalp for *at least* 2 hours before you shampoo.

- Whisk 1 teaspoon of ground black pepper (*or* the juice of 1 lemon) into ½ a cup of plain yogurt. Massage this mixture onto your scalp and leave it on for approximately 20 minutes before you shampoo. This application not only slows down the process of graying, but also leaves your hair feeling soft. Employ this remedy once a week. (Note: Allow the yogurt to warm to room temperature before you apply this mixture—applying cold yogurt could cause a headache.)

- Two-to-three times a week, massage your scalp for approximately 10 minutes with a mixture made from 1 part of lemon juice and 2 parts of warm coconut oil. Leave this on for *at least* 1 hour before you shampoo. This remedy is also effective for treating dandruff. (Note: Do not sit out in the sun or use any heated appliances, such as a blow dryer, while you have this application on—combined with heat, lemon juice is known to impart highlights to hair.)

PREMATURE GRAYING

- Heat 5 fluid ounces of coconut oil on a stovetop. Once moderately hot, add to it 3.5 ounces of curry leaves. Let these cook in the oil on low-to-medium heat until they turn black. (This will also cause the color of the oil to change.) Once the concoction has cooled, strain the oil and preserve it in a container for future use. *At least* once a week, if not more often, apply it onto your hair and scalp before you go to bed. Leave it on overnight.

Hair Loss

- Before you go to bed, massage onto your scalp some warm castor oil. Shampoo your hair the following morning. Try to employ this remedy *at least* once a week, if not more often.

- Soak a cotton pad in some lemon juice and dab it onto the thinning areas of your scalp. Leave this on for approximately 30 minutes before you shampoo. (Note: Do not sit out in the sun or use any heated appliances, such as a blow dryer, while you have on the lemon juice application—combined with heat, lemon juice is known to impart highlights to hair.)

- As regularly as time permits, each time before you shampoo, massage onto your hair and scalp a warm mixture of equal quantities of mustard and almond oils. Leave this on for *at least* 1 hour, in order to give the oils a chance to absorb. This remedy is effective for treating both hair loss and dandruff.

- Gooseberry makes an excellent remedy for hair loss. It also helps cure other scalp and hair-related problems, such as dandruff, dull or dry hair, and premature graying. Mix 1 teaspoon of gooseberry powder with some warm olive, coconut, *or* almond oil and apply this paste onto your scalp for *at least* 2 hours before you shampoo.

HAIR LOSS

- Oils like gooseberry and neem do wonders for our hair. Like any other oil, massage either of these gently onto your hair and scalp. Leave it on for *at least* 1 hour before you shampoo. These oils are very effective for treating hair loss, dandruff, and dull or dry hair.

- To prevent hair loss, mix 1 raw egg with just enough olive oil to give you good coverage on your hair and scalp; apply this mixture and leave it on for *at least* 1 hour before you shampoo. (Note: Beware of rinsing your hair in hot water—the egg could scramble and become difficult to tease out!)

- If you suffer from thinning hair or baldness, apply onto your scalp a soft paste made from warm olive oil, 1 tablespoon of honey, and 1 teaspoon of cinnamon powder. Leave this on for approximately 30 minutes before you shampoo.

- Soak equal quantities of gooseberry and henna powders in just enough water to form a moderately thick paste. Instead of your usual shampoo, wash your hair with this mixture. Rinse with your regular conditioner. This remedy not only promotes hair growth, but also softens your hair and infuses the shine back into it. (Note: Henna imparts a rich, brownish-red color to black or brunette hair. Its use also stains our skin, so make sure that you use a pair of gloves when you employ this remedy.)

HAIR LOSS

- Yogurt contains all the elements that our hair needs in order to be healthy. Apply some mashed, plain yogurt onto your scalp and leave it on for 20–30 minutes before you shampoo. This remedy not only reduces hair loss, but also makes your hair soft. (Note: Allow the yogurt to warm to room temperature before you apply it—applying cold yogurt could cause a headache.)

- Whenever you have a few moments, seize the opportunity to massage your scalp vigorously. This increases the circulation of blood to your head and activates your sebaceous (oil) glands, stimulating them to produce your own natural oils.

Dandruff

Simply explained, dandruff is nothing but dry skin that flakes off your scalp, usually causing itchiness. This condition commonly bares itself in dry weather. The key is to infuse and retain moisture in your scalp, otherwise, you will not only find yourself dealing with dandruff, but also, your hair will not have a healthy base, which could further result in hair loss. (Think of this using soil and plants as examples—if the soil is not nourished with moisture, the plants that grow in it will have nothing on which to survive.) So, give your scalp the regular attention it deserves…it is also, after all, a part of your skin.

- Before you go to bed, massage onto your scalp some warm coconut (*or* almond) oil. This remedy successfully counteracts dryness.

- Gooseberry makes an excellent remedy for dandruff. It also helps cure other scalp and hair-related problems, such as hair loss, dull or dry hair, and premature graying. Mix 1 teaspoon of gooseberry powder with some warm olive, coconut, *or* almond oil and apply this paste onto your scalp for *at least* 2 hours before you shampoo.

- Whisk 1 egg in a bowl. Rinse your hair with water, and then massage the beaten egg onto your scalp. Leave it on for 3–5 minutes. Rinse again, until your hair is no longer slick. (Note: Beware of rinsing your hair in hot water—the egg could scramble and become difficult to tease out!)

DANDRUFF

- Mix 1 part of lemon juice with 2 parts of warm coconut oil. Massage this mixture onto your scalp. Leave it on for *at least* 1 hour before you shampoo. This remedy also effectively treats premature graying. (Note: Do not sit out in the sun or use any heated appliances, such as a blow dryer, while you have this application on—combined with heat, lemon juice is known to impart highlights to hair.)

- As regularly as time permits, each time before you shampoo, massage onto your scalp a warm mixture of equal quantities of mustard and almond oils. Leave this on for *at least* 1 hour, in order to give the oils a chance to absorb. This remedy is effective for treating both dandruff and hair loss.

- Mix together 4 tablespoons of gram flour and 1 tablespoon of apple cider vinegar. Add water as needed to form a paste of medium-to-thick consistency. Apply this mixture onto your scalp and leave it on for approximately 30 minutes before you shampoo.

- Oils like gooseberry and neem do wonders for our hair. Like any other oil, massage either of these gently onto your hair and scalp. Leave it on for *at least* 1 hour before you shampoo. These oils are very effective for treating dandruff, hair loss, and dull or dry hair.

- Add 3 tablespoons of lemon juice (*or* 3 tablespoons of apple cider vinegar) to 1 cup of warm water. After you shampoo, rinse your hair

DANDRUFF

with either mixture. Both lemon juice and vinegar not only effectively treat dandruff, but also dissolve excess oil deposits on your scalp, infuse the shine back into dull or dry hair, and strip out any shampoo or styling product residue from your strands. (Note: While vinegar is known to add highlights to brunette hair, combined with heat, lemon juice also imparts highlights to hair. If you use the lemon juice mixture, let your hair dry naturally—do not sit out in the sun or use any heated appliances, such as a blow dryer.)

- Whisk 1 teaspoon of kitchen salt into 1 cup of plain yogurt. Massage this mixture onto your scalp. Leave it on for 20-30 minutes, and then rinse your hair with plain water. Employ this remedy once a week. (Note: Allow the yogurt to warm to room temperature before you apply this mixture—applying cold yogurt could cause a headache.)

Shampoo and Styling Product Build-Up

- Add 3 tablespoons of lemon juice (*or* 3 tablespoons of apple cider vinegar) to 1 cup of warm water. After you shampoo, soak your hair well with either mixture. Leave it on for approximately 5 minutes, and then rinse it off with tolerably cool water. (In the alternative, add 4–5 drops of lemon juice *or* 4–5 drops of apple cider vinegar directly to your dollop of shampoo—massage this mixture onto your hair and scalp, and then rinse it off as you normally would.) Both lemon juice and vinegar not only strip out any shampoo and styling product residue from your strands, but also effectively treat oily hair, dull or dry hair, and dandruff. (Note: While vinegar is known to add highlights to brunette hair, combined with heat, lemon juice also imparts highlights to hair. If you use the lemon juice mixture, let your hair dry naturally—do not sit out in the sun or use any heated appliances, such as a blow dryer.)

EYES

Considered as the most expressive of all our features, our eyes are also the most developed of all our sensory organs. They are especially delicate and warrant gentle care. Also very delicate is the skin that surrounds them, and not caring for it properly leads to premature fine lines and wrinkles around our eyes that are commonly referred to as crow's feet.

In looking for eye makeup, you will find a barrage of products to enhance your eyes—eye shadow, eyeliner, mascara, eyebrow pencils, false eyelashes, and under-eye concealers, to name just a few. While there is absolutely nothing wrong with trying to make your eyes look as attractive as possible, if the thought of cleansing off your makeup and revealing what's underneath worries you, you can fall back on the following home remedies to overcome some of the most common problems that you might be experiencing.

(Note: For remedies on ***Premature Aging*** and ***Fine Lines and Wrinkles***, please refer to the "**FACE**" section in this book.)

Eyebrows and Eyelashes

- To thicken your eyebrows, use your fingertip to blend into them a mixture of a drop each of glycerin and *pure* castor oil. Do this daily before you go to bed, leaving the application on overnight. Employ this remedy for *at least* six weeks to see results.

- To thicken and lengthen your eyelashes, use your fore-fingertips to gently coat them with a drop of *pure* castor oil, making sure that you cover the base areas. Do this daily before you go to bed, leaving the application on overnight. Employ this remedy for approximately three months to see results. (Note: Using this remedy on your eyelashes may cause a bit of the oil to enter your eyes—this is not harmful; on the contrary, it cleanses your eyes. However, if you are allergic, or are unsure of any allergies, to castor oil, *do not* employ this remedy.)

- If you use an eyelash curler, you have probably experienced that to provide the effect that it does, if not clasped properly, it pulls out an eyelash or two or even pinches the delicate skin on your eyelids. A safe, yet effective, eyelash curler is none other than your own fingertip. Before you apply your mascara, using your fore-fingertips, gently press down your eyelashes in 3-second spurts with them pointed in the upward direction. Do this from corner-to-corner of each eye. (Note: In employing this remedy, make sure that you avoid pressing down too hard on your eyes.)

Tired Eyes

- Place a cool slice of an unpeeled cucumber on each eye. Lay back and relax for approximately 20 minutes. This remedy also effectively treats puffy eyes and dark circles.

- Soak two cotton pads in cold milk. Place one on each eye and leave them on for 10–15 minutes.

- Mix 2–3 drops of castor oil (*or* 2–3 drops of fresh lemon juice) in a little rosewater. Soak two cotton pads in this mixture and place them on your eyelids. Lay back and relax for 15–20 minutes.

- Get into the habit of beginning and ending your day by gently splashing your open eyes with cool water. This will not only thoroughly cleanse them, but also stimulate them.

- Did you know that crying is good for your eyes? Our tears are the most natural and effective cleansers for our eyes; so, for those of you that have been holding them back, bawl away!

Puffy Eyes

- Add 4 drops of rosewater to 2 tablespoons of cold milk (*or* 4 drops of Vitamin E oil to 2 tablespoons of cold rosewater). Soak two cotton pads in either mixture and place them on your eyelids. Lay back and relax for 15–20 minutes.

- To reduce the bags under your eyes, add a ¼ teaspoon of kitchen salt to 4 tablespoons of warm water. Soak two cotton pads in this mixture and place them on your eyes for 5–7 minutes. Once the cotton pads have cooled, soak them once again in the remaining warm saltwater mixture and place them back on your eyes for another 5–7 minutes.

- Cut out two slices of a raw potato. Place one slice on each eye. Lay back and relax for 15–20 minutes.

- Whisk the white of an egg in a bowl. Use a cotton pad to evenly smooth this onto the skin around your eyes; leave it on until the egg white begins to tighten. Use a cotton pad soaked in milk to gently cleanse it off, finally rinsing your skin with tolerably cold water.

- Place a thin, cool slice of an unpeeled cucumber on each eye. Lay back and relax for approximately 20 minutes. This remedy is also effective for treating dark circles and tired eyes.

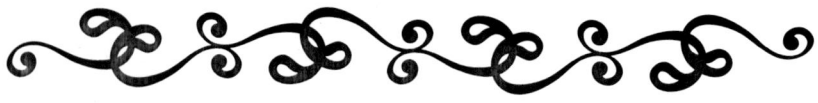

PUFFY EYES

- Apply a few drops of castor oil around your eyes before you go to bed. (Plastic surgeons use this remedy very effectively on their patients after surgery.)

Dark Circles

- Smooth a few drops of almond, coconut, sesame *or* Vitamin E oil around your eyes before you go to bed each night.

- To reduce the appearance of dark circles, place a cool slice of an unpeeled cucumber on each eye. Lay back and relax for approximately 20 minutes. This remedy is also effective for treating tired or puffy eyes.

- Mix ½ a teaspoon of a pureed tomato with a pinch of turmeric powder and a ¼ teaspoon each of lemon juice and gram flour. Apply this onto the dark circles under your eyes and leave it on until it begins to dry. Use a cotton pad soaked in milk to gently cleanse the application off, finally rinsing your skin with tolerably cold water.

- Before you go to bed each night, use your fore-fingertip to apply a small amount of mashed clotted cream onto your dark circles. Leave this on overnight. Rinse it off the next morning using lukewarm water.

- Grate a small piece each of a raw potato and cucumber, both unpeeled. Mix the resulting shreds together. Use your hand or a fine strainer to extract their juice. Soak two cotton pads in this mixture and place one over each eye. This remedy not only reduces the appearance of dark circles, but also tones and refreshes the skin around your eyes.

DARK CIRCLES

- Mix together a ¼ teaspoon each of yogurt and honey. Smooth this onto the dark circles under your eyes. Leave it on for approximately 15 minutes, and then rinse it off with tolerably cold water.

- Form a paste by crushing 1 teaspoon's worth of fresh basil leaves (*or* 1 teaspoon's worth of fresh mint leaves). Add to this a ¼ teaspoon of rosewater. Apply this mixture onto your dark circles and leave it on for 15–20 minutes. Rinse it off with tolerably cold water.

FACE

Many of us have, at one time or another, envied glamorous models on TV or in print for their watertight skin and radiant glow; our eyes have scanned their faces for that *one* imperfection, only to leave us disappointed. We have wondered during these moments about how much time and care they must invest in themselves, or how expensive the skin care products they use might be, in order for them to have attained that level of flawlessness. It seems impossible that any of us would achieve those results, given that most of us are on shoestring budgets and our days don't have enough hours in them for us to be able to spend that kind of time on ourselves.

If you admittedly fall in the category of people above, you are definitely not alone. Our skin, especially facial, is a constant source of worry for many of us. It depicts the story of how we are affected by the changes in our physical or emotional environments. Factors that affect us include, but are not limited to, excess stress, work and strain, irregular sleeping and eating habits, the weather, etc. Additionally, foods that contain artificial flavors, colors, preservatives, and chemicals also accelerate the process of skin degeneration. Before we've even achieved the wisdom to appreciate the flawless texture of the skin we

had as babies, we find ourselves facing teenage skin problems, and by the time we overcome *those,* we are left to battle the aging process head-on.

While aging is a natural phenomenon that we cannot avoid, we can, however, delay it. It is *never too early,* and it's certainly *never too late* to begin maintaining, preserving, and even repairing your skin. In taking steps to accomplish these, it is important to know that there are two kinds of aging:

1. *Intrinsic (Internal) Aging*—This form of aging is controlled by the genes we inherit. With the natural passage of time, our skin inevitably gets thinner. We increasingly lose collagen and elastin, the two proteins mainly responsible for the firmness and moisture in our skin. The good news is that intrinsic aging contributes to only 10–20% of the aging process and is regarded as the graceful way to age. The solution to minimize the effects of this kind of aging is as simple as this—Moisturize! Moisturize! Moisturize!

2. *Extrinsic (External) Aging*—This form of aging cumulatively occurs as a result of the constant surge of abuse that our skin faces from factors such as excessive exposure to the sun, pollution, and chemically-formulated products, *or* neglect due to an unhealthy lifestyle. These factors continually strip our skin of its natural balance and are responsible for a staggering 80–90% of the aging process. The good

news in the case of extrinsic aging is that there are several ways to minimize its onset or even recover from its effects—do recognize that the personal choices you make today will *definitely* reflect on your skin in the years to come.

There are five main skin types—oily, dry, combination, normal, and sensitive. Each skin type has different needs, and it is important to know what skin type you have. Once you've determined this, the secret to an all-encompassing healthy complexion is to get into a regular beauty routine—stick with the aid you decide to employ, however being a little adventurous from time-to-time and exercising your flexibility to use varying natural ingredients. Also, incorporate these basics into your routine—they will go a very long way:

❋ Drink enough water—water not only cleanses your body of toxins, but also acts as an internal moisturizer for it, helping your skin retain its natural essential oils that shield it against dryness.

❋ Moisturize *at least* once each day, even if you have oily skin, (or even if you belong to the male species!).

❋ Use a sunblock lotion (*or* moisturizer) that contains an ultraviolet (UV) ray protectant with a Sun Protection Factor (SPF) of *at least* 15 or more. (Note, however, that higher the SPF, longer the protection.)

❋ *Always* cleanse your skin before you go to bed.

NOTE

In employing any remedy throughout this section, *always* use tolerably cold water to rinse it off, unless you've used any oil as an ingredient when concocting it, in which case, you should use lukewarm water for your final rinse—cold water tightens your pores, sealing in the nourishment from the ingredients that you used, whereas lukewarm water works best to gently dissolve and cleanse any excess oil left on your skin after an application.

Oily Skin

Before you use any of these remedies, make sure that you read the **NOTE** *on Page* 34.

- The best astringent for an oily complexion is a ¼ teaspoon of lemon juice mixed in with 1 teaspoon each of rosewater and cucumber juice. Using these proportions, you can concoct a slightly larger quantity of this mixture and store it in the fridge for your daily cleansing routine before bed.

- Mix together 2 tablespoons of fuller's earth, ½ a tablespoon of sandalwood powder, and just enough rosewater to form a paste. Apply this mask onto your skin and leave it on until it begins to dry.

- Gently rub the inside of a lemon rind on your face—this will not only neutralize the oil on your skin, but also lighten your complexion. Rinse your skin after approximately 5 minutes, and then pat on a light layer of oil-free moisturizer.

- Rub the inside of a papaya peel on your face, allowing its juice to wet your skin. Leave it on for *no more than* 5–10 minutes. (You can also use a mixture of 2 tablespoons of mashed papaya pulp and a few drops of lemon juice.)

OILY SKIN

- Grate ½ an unpeeled apple. Place the resulting shreds on your skin. Sit back and relax for approximately 15 minutes. (If you don't have an apple at home, use some bottled apple juice instead.)

- Whisk together 1 egg white, ½ a teaspoon of honey, and a few drops of lemon juice. Apply this onto your skin and leave it on for 25–30 minutes. Use a cotton pad soaked in cold milk to cleanse the mask off, finally rinsing your skin with water.

- Mix 1 tablespoon of tomato puree (*or* 1 tablespoon of plain yogurt) with ½ a teaspoon of sandalwood powder and a few drops of lemon juice. Apply this pack onto your skin and leave it on for 20–25 minutes.

- The best way to care for oily skin is to cleanse it twice a day using lukewarm water and a cream-based cleanser, both of which effectively dissolve any excess oil on your skin. You definitely want to stay away from soap-based cleansers, which strip your skin of even that oil which is necessary to keep it from becoming dry. After cleansing, use an oil-free moisturizer to ensure that your skin stays shine-free and yet supple.

Dry Skin

Before you use any of these remedies, make sure that you read the **NOTE** *on Page* 34.

- Whisk the juice of ½ a lemon with 2 teaspoons of olive oil and the yolk of an egg. Apply this mask and leave it on until it begins to tighten on your skin.

- Whisk 1 egg with ½ a teaspoon each of honey, glycerin, and almond oil. Apply this mask and leave it on for 20–30 minutes.

- Mix together 1 teaspoon each of honey, olive oil, orange juice, and rosewater. Apply this onto your face and neck, and leave it on for approximately 25 minutes.

- Whisk 1 tablespoon each of rosewater and milk with 1 egg yolk. Apply this onto your skin and leave it on for approximately 30 minutes. Use a cotton pad soaked in milk to cleanse the mask off, finally rinsing your skin with water.

- Mix 1 tablespoon each of sandalwood and neem powders with just enough rosewater to form a paste. (If you don't have rosewater at home, you can also use the juice from a small piece of grated cucumber *or* from a few hand-squeezed seedless green grapes.) Apply this mixture onto your

DRY SKIN

skin and leave it on until it begins to dry. Employ this remedy daily, until you see results. Over and above infusing moisture and softening dry skin, this pack also makes an effective remedy for pimples and acne.

- Before you go to bed, massage onto your skin just enough coconut oil so that it absorbs, followed by a few drops of glycerin to seal in the moisture.

- Mix together 1 tablespoon each of honey and almond powder. Apply this onto your skin and leave it on for 15–20 minutes. Dip your fingertips in some cold milk and then employ them in circular motions to gently loosen the mask, finally rinsing your skin with water. (Note: Make sure that you do not over-exfoliate—30 seconds should suffice.)

- Blend to a smooth pulp ½ a ripe banana and 1 tablespoon of rosewater. Use this facemask once a week for approximately 30 minutes.

- Mix together 1 teaspoon each of gram flour, honey, and clotted cream. Add a ¼ teaspoon of turmeric powder and a few drops of lemon juice. Apply this mask and leave it on until it begins to dry.

- Make it a habit to moisturize your skin *everyday*—no exceptions! Preferably, use your moisturizer on damp skin, for example, when you've just come out of the shower or after you've just washed your face. This will increase the moisture on the outer layers of your skin.

Dark or Dull Complexion

Before you use any of these remedies, make sure that you read the **NOTE** *on Page* 34.

- One of the most natural bleaches for your skin is a mixture made from the juice of 1 lemon and 2 tablespoons of clotted cream (*or 2* tablespoons of cold milk). Using your fingertips, massage either mixture onto your skin in circular motions, *after* you have cleansed your face before bed each night. Do this for a few minutes. Rinse your skin with water, and then apply your bedtime moisturizer.

- Gently rub the inside of a lemon rind on your face. Rinse your skin after approximately 5 minutes, and then pat on a light layer of moisturizer. This remedy not only lightens your complexion, but also restores the moisture balance on oily skin.

- Mix together 1 tablespoon each of cucumber juice and lemon juice. Add to this a ¼ teaspoon of turmeric powder. Using a cotton pad, evenly apply this mixture onto your face and neck. Leave it on for approximately 30 minutes. This lotion not only lightens your complexion, but also makes an excellent astringent.

- Mix 1 teaspoon of lemon juice with ½ a teaspoon each of honey and milk. Apply this mixture onto your skin to lighten your complexion.

DARK OR DULL COMPLEXION

- Mix 1 tablespoon of gram flour with 1 teaspoon each of plain yogurt and freshly pureed tomato pulp, ½ a teaspoon of lemon juice, and a ¼ teaspoon of turmeric powder. Apply this onto your face and neck, and leave it on for 20–25 minutes.

- Cut a tomato in half. Using circular motions, gently scrub your face and neck with its insides. This remedy not only lightens your skin, but also tones and refines your pores.

- Using circular motions, gently massage onto your skin a slice or two of a raw potato.

- Mix 1 teaspoon of gram flour with a ¼ teaspoon of turmeric powder. Add ½ a teaspoon each of olive oil and milk, and 4–5 drops of lemon juice. Apply this onto your skin and leave it on for 25–30 minutes.

- Mix 2 teaspoons of turmeric powder with just enough milk to form a paste. Apply this evenly onto your face and neck. Leave it on until it begins to dry. This remedy not only helps to lighten your complexion, but also stops the growth of superfluous hair on your face. (Note: Due to turmeric's tendency to lend its color when applied, make sure that you keep this mixture out of contact with your hairline. On the other

DARK OR DULL COMPLEXION

hand, if you find that your *skin* has absorbed some color, simply use a cotton pad soaked in milk to cleanse it out.)

- To treat sunburn, mix 1 teaspoon of lemon juice with a ¼ cup of milk. (Depending on your need for coverage, adjust the quantity of these ingredients in the proportions listed.) Using a cotton pad, gently and evenly dab this mixture onto the affected areas. Leave it on for approximately 20 minutes before you shower.

- Another remedy to treat sunburn is to blend ¼ of an unpeeled cucumber with 4 tablespoons each of rosewater and glycerin. Using a fine strainer, filter out the resulting liquid mixture. Before you shower, apply this onto the affected areas and leave it on for 15–20 minutes.

- Also effective for sunburn is a moderately thick paste made from fuller's earth and sesame (*or* coconut) oil. Spread this evenly onto the affected areas and leave it on for 20–25 minutes before you shower.

Uneven Pigmentation

Before you use any of these remedies, make sure that you read the **NOTE** *on Page* 34.

- Mix a few drops of lemon juice with 1 teaspoon each of almond powder and clotted cream. Apply this onto the affected areas. Leave it on for approximately 15 minutes.

- Once a week, evenly apply some papaya juice (*or* some mashed papaya pulp) onto the affected areas of your skin, leaving it on for *no more than* 5–10 minutes.

- Grind together 1 teaspoon each of sesame seeds and turmeric powder, and just enough rosewater to form a paste. Apply this onto the discolored areas of your skin. Rinse it off once the mask begins to dry. (Note: Due to turmeric's tendency to lend its color when applied, make sure that you keep this mixture out of contact with your hairline. On the other hand, if you find that your *skin* has absorbed some color, simply use a cotton pad soaked in milk to cleanse it out.)

- Whisk 2–3 drops of lemon juice with 1 teaspoon of yogurt. Apply this onto the affected areas and leave it on for approximately 30 minutes.

UNEVEN PIGMENTATION

- Form a paste by crushing a few fresh basil leaves (*or* a few fresh mint leaves). Add to this 1 tablespoon each of lemon juice and rosewater. As regularly as time permits, apply this onto the discolored areas of your skin.

- If you're battling with uneven pigmentation, especially protect your skin from excessive exposure to the sun.

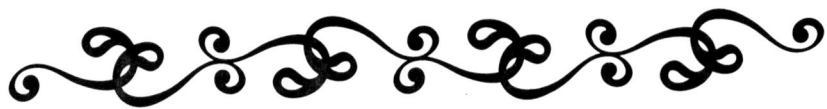

Freckles

Before you use any of these remedies, make sure that you read the **NOTE** *on Page 34.*

- While you can't completely eliminate freckles, you can certainly reduce their appearance. Add 1 teaspoon of lemon juice to 1 tablespoon of buttermilk (*or* 1 tablespoon of rosewater). Soak a cotton pad in either mixture and dab it onto your freckles. Leave it on until it dries.

- Reduce the appearance of your freckles by gently massaging onto them a slice of a freshly cut eggplant. Employ this remedy everyday, until you see results.

- Cut out a thin slice of a raw potato and dip it in buttermilk. Gently massage it onto your freckles. Employ this remedy 3–4 times a week.

- Grate a small piece of a cucumber. Use your hand or a fine strainer to squeeze out the equivalent of 1 tablespoon of its juice. Mix into it 1 teaspoon of lemon juice and a ¼ teaspoon of fuller's earth. Using a cotton pad, dab this mixture evenly onto your freckles. Leave it on until it dries.

- Puree ¼ of a tomato in a mini blender. Use a cotton pad to evenly apply the pulp onto the affected areas. Leave it on for approximately 20 minutes.

Clogged Pores and Blackheads

Blackheads develop not only on our faces, but also on other areas of our body that are rich in sebaceous (oil) glands. While most of us know what blackheads are, many of us are unaware of how they form through their correlation with clogged pores. The following is a basic explanation: overactive oil glands in our skin secrete excess oil through their surrounding pores, causing them to expand. The oil then begins to accumulate in these expanded pores, eventually hardening into plugs. The presence of these plugs further enlarges the affected pores, exposing the plugs' tips to the air, thereby causing them to oxidize (turn black). The black-tip appearance of these plugs is the very reason that they came to be termed as "blackheads."

From the above explanation, it becomes apparent that those who have blackheads usually have an oily skin type. Taking on a domino effect, the oil present on the surface of their skin tends to adhere to the dirt and grime in the air. These pollutants, in turn, seep into their pores and exacerbate existing blackheads, causing their skin texture to become coarse over time, *if* they neglect the presence of those blackheads.

Blackheads not only clog our pores, but also rob the skin that surrounds these clogged pores of precious oxygen. This further makes those affected areas of our skin susceptible to infections that surface in the form of pimples and acne. It is

CLOGGED PORES AND BLACKHEADS

therefore very important that we keep our pores clean, in order to prevent the domino effect described above. Employing the following remedies will help you accomplish this.

Before you use any of these remedies, make sure that you read the **NOTE** *on Page* 34.

- Mix 3 tablespoons of plain yogurt with 2 tablespoons of grated orange peel. Using circular motions, gently exfoliate your skin with this mixture for 4–5 minutes. (Note: The orange rind might make your skin tingle.)

- Once a day, soak a cotton pad in some lemon juice and dab it onto the affected areas. Leave it on for approximately 5 minutes. After you rinse it off, make sure that you then pat a small amount of an oil-free moisturizer onto your skin. (Note: Lemon juice is a potent astringent—if you have a dry skin type, dilute the lemon juice in some rosewater before dabbing it on.)

- Mix together 1 tablespoon of gram flour (*or* 1 tablespoon of almond powder), 1 teaspoon of honey, ½ a teaspoon of sandalwood powder, and just enough rosewater to form a soft paste. Apply this mask evenly onto your skin, paying special attention to any blackhead-cluttered areas. Leave it on for 15–20 minutes.

CLOGGED PORES AND BLACKHEADS

- Mix together 1 tablespoon each of gram flour, plain yogurt, lemon juice, and olive oil. Apply this paste onto your skin. Leave it on for 10–15 minutes.

- To help prevent the blockage of pores, always make sure that your skin is absolutely clean before you apply any makeup. Further, before you go to bed each night, cleanse your skin of all makeup. (Our skin cells repair themselves while we're asleep, and any blocked pores only hinder this process.)

- To discourage the occurrence of blackheads, tighten your pores by using a cotton pad to smooth a whisked egg white onto your skin. Leave it on for approximately 15 minutes.

- Squeeze the juice out of a small piece of watermelon. Using a cotton pad, dab this onto your skin and leave it on for approximately 15 minutes. Rinse it off with lukewarm water first, and then with tolerably cold water. This remedy not only tones your skin, but also clears it of blemishes.

- Another effective toner is none other than an ice-cube. Glide an ice-cube or two against your skin, preferably after a facemask. This tightens your pores *and* increases the blood circulation to those areas. (If you have an

CLOGGED PORES AND BLACKHEADS

ice-cube tray at home, ice-cubes made using rosewater are even more effective as skin toners—in addition to benefiting you as described above, they leave your skin feeling petal-soft.)

Pimples, Acne, and Blemishes

As mentioned in the "***Clogged Pores and Blackheads***" section, when our pores are clogged with blackheads, the skin that surrounds those clogged pores is robbed of precious oxygen, which makes it susceptible to infections that surface in the form of pimples and acne. Pimples and acne, in turn, leave behind skin discolorations or scars that are commonly known as blemishes. You can prevent this logical progression that yields blemished skin by keeping your pores clean. Remember—Prevention *is* Better than Cure!

The remedies in this section will help you cleanse and clarify your skin. If you have a severe occurrence of pimples and acne, apply your chosen remedy for longer than suggested, for example, overnight, if possible.

Before you use any of these remedies, make sure that you read the **NOTE** *on Page* 34.

- Mix 1 tablespoon of gram flour with just enough cucumber (*or* carrot) juice to form a thick paste. Apply this evenly onto the affected areas of your skin. Leave it on until it begins to dry.

- Mix together 1 teaspoon each of gram flour and lemon juice. Add to this mixture a ¼ teaspoon of turmeric powder and just enough rosewater to form a paste. Apply this onto your skin and leave it on until it begins to dry.

PIMPLES, ACNE, AND BLEMISHES

- Mix together equal quantities each of cucumber juice (*or* glycerin), lemon juice, and rosewater. Using a cotton pad, dab this mixture onto your skin. Leave it on for 30–45 minutes. Employ this remedy as regularly as time permits—it will not only clarify your complexion, but also help it stay that way. This remedy can also be effectively used on the rest of your body to reduce the appearance of scars and blemishes.

- Blend together 1 tablespoon of gram flour (*or* 1 tablespoon of sandalwood powder), ½ a teaspoon of turmeric powder, 1 teaspoon's worth of a banana, and just enough milk to form a paste. Apply this onto the affected areas and leave it on until it begins to dry.

- Mix together 1 tablespoon each of grated orange rind, plain yogurt, and rosewater. Apply this pack onto your skin and leave it on for approximately 20 minutes. (Note: The orange rind might make your skin tingle.)

- Mix 1 tablespoon each of sandalwood and neem powders with just enough rosewater to form a paste. (If you don't have rosewater at home, you can also use the juice from a small piece of grated cucumber *or* from a few hand-squeezed seedless green grapes.) Apply this mixture onto the affected areas of your skin and leave it on until it begins to dry. Employ this remedy daily, until your skin has cleared. Over and above

PIMPLES, ACNE, AND BLEMISHES

warding off pimples and acne, this pack effectively infuses moisture into dry skin, leaving it feeling soft and supple.

- Form a paste by mixing 2 tablespoons of honey with 2 teaspoons of cinnamon powder. Apply this onto the affected areas of your skin and leave it on for *at least* 1 hour, if not longer. Use this remedy daily for three weeks. If your acne is deep-rooted, continue to employ this remedy until your skin clears. (Note: During the first three-to-four applications, you will feel a hot and tingly sensation on your skin; ride it out if you can—it is none other than the medicinal power of the cinnamon powder working on your skin—this sensation will subside gradually. Furthermore, if your pimples and acne worsen at first, don't panic—this concoction is known to penetrate your pores and draw out any impurities—your skin will show signs of improvement with each successive application.)

- Using a cotton pad, dab some aloe vera (*or* pineapple) juice onto the affected areas of your skin. Leave it on for 20–30 minutes.

- Mix ½ a teaspoon of turmeric powder with just enough coconut (*or* sesame) oil to form a paste. Apply this mixture onto the affected areas of your skin and leave it on for approximately 20 minutes. (Note: Due to turmeric's tendency to lend its color when applied, make sure that you

PIMPLES, ACNE, AND BLEMISHES

keep this mixture out of contact with your hairline. On the other hand, if you find that your *skin* has absorbed some color, simply use a cotton pad soaked in milk to cleanse it out.)

- Mix together 1 teaspoon of cumin powder and just enough plain yogurt to form a paste. Apply this evenly onto your skin and leave it on for approximately 45 minutes.

- Crush 4 tablespoon's worth of fresh mint leaves. Add to this 1 tablespoon of gram flour and just enough rosewater to form a paste. Apply this onto your face and neck, and leave it on until it begins to dry.

- Using a cotton pad, dab some lemon juice onto the affected areas of your skin. Leave it on for approximately 5 minutes. Employ this remedy daily, until your skin clears. (Note: Lemon juice is a potent astringent—if you have a dry skin type, make sure that you dilute the lemon juice in some rosewater before dabbing it on.)

- Nourish your face *at least* once a week using a mixture made from 1 tablespoon of fuller's earth, a ¼ teaspoon each of turmeric and sandalwood powders, 4–5 drops of lemon juice, and just enough rosewater to form a paste. Leave it on until it begins to dry.

PIMPLES, ACNE, AND BLEMISHES

- Blend to a smooth pulp ¼ of an unpeeled apple and 3 teaspoons of honey. Apply this mask evenly onto the affected areas of your skin and leave it on for approximately 20 minutes.

- Squeeze the juice out of a small piece of watermelon. Using a cotton pad, dab this onto your skin and leave it on for approximately 15 minutes. Rinse it off with lukewarm water first, and then with tolerably cold water. This remedy not only clears your skin of blemishes, but also tones and refreshes it.

- To reduce the appearance of blemishes, mix together 1 tablespoon each of sandalwood powder, yogurt, and honey. Apply this mixture onto the affected areas and leave it on for 40–45 minutes.

- Reduce the appearance of blemishes or any redness that surrounds your pimples by firmly holding a slice of a raw potato against the affected areas of your skin for approximately 10 minutes.

- Another remedy for reducing the appearance of blemishes is to crush a teaspoon's worth of fresh basil leaves (*or* a teaspoon's worth of fresh mint leaves); then add to this paste 1 tablespoon of honey and 4–5 drops of lemon juice. Apply this mixture onto the affected areas and leave

PIMPLES, ACNE, AND BLEMISHES

it on for approximately 20 minutes. This remedy not only aids in reducing the appearance of blemishes, but also lends your complexion a healthy glow.

- If you find that you are breaking out around your eyes or on your eyelids, smear a drop of refined castor oil onto the affected areas before you go to bed each night.

- Always cleanse your facial skin with cream-based cleansers or with milk, and never soap or soap-based cleansers. (You can identify the latter by their foam.) While soap-based cleansers are effective in cleaning your face, they tend to go one step further by stripping your skin of your own natural oils. Cream-based cleansers, on the other hand, are just as effective, but don't rob your skin of these essential oils.

- Honey is amazingly curative in healing blemishes and scars—add a teaspoon of it to any of the remedies above!

Premature Aging

Before you use any of these remedies, make sure that you read the **NOTE** *on Page* 34.

- One of the best beauty treatments for your skin is none other than plain water. All you have to do is to consume as much as your body needs, otherwise, you will be depriving yourself of the least expensive anti-aging treatment!

- Before you go to bed each night, gently massage a few drops of almond, olive, sesame, *or* coconut oil onto your face and neck, using circular motions on your face and upward strokes on your neck.

- To reduce the appearance of age spots on your face or body, massage a few drops of Vitamin E oil onto your skin before you go to bed each night. This remedy is also effective for ironing out the fine lines around your eyes.

- The sun's rays have a direct and adverse effect on our skin cells. They cause our skin to shrivel in the same way that fresh fruit does, when it loses its moisture. For those of you that spend a good bit of your time outdoors, whether working or exercising, expect approximately a 20% reduction in your collagen levels in your lifetime due to your day-to-day sun exposure. (Bear in mind that this does *not* account for those of you who worship the sun to satisfy your obsession for that perfectly bronzed tan—you need to recognize that the sun is high up on the list

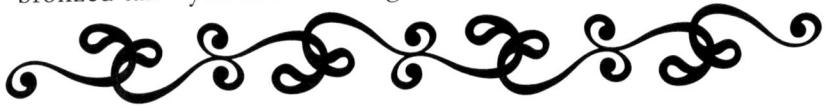

PREMATURE AGING

among the external factors that are responsible for 80–90% of our skin's aging—so, think about *that* the next time you decide to bathe in it!)

- To treat sun-damaged skin, coarsely grind 4 tablespoon's worth of papaya seeds in a mini blender. (If you don't have a papaya at home, you can also use bottled papaya juice.) Apply this onto the affected areas and leave it on for *no more than* 5–10 minutes. Employ this remedy once a week.

- Assuming that we get the recommended 8 hours of sleep each night, we spend one-third of our lives sleeping; to put this fact into perspective, by age 60, the average person will have slept for twenty years! With that amount of time spent on our pillows, the formation of sleep wrinkles—the facial creases that develop from sleeping with our face against a pillow—becomes inevitable. As we age, these wrinkles prominently etch themselves in our skin. The good news is that they can be prevented. The easiest way to achieve this is by making an effort to sleep on your back. If you are unable to do so, however, either use a fluffy pillow *or* slip a silk or satin pillowcase onto your pillow—both of these effectively aid in minimizing the onset of sleep wrinkles.

- Don't underestimate the extent to which our facial expressions contribute to the formation of furrows and crow's feet on our skin. It is common

PREMATURE AGING

knowledge that it takes only 14 muscles to smile, but over 70 muscles to frown. So smile more, and find yourself age less!

- As we age, our bones shrink *and* we increasingly lose the fat that underlies our skin. The resulting loose skin gradually surrenders to gravity, causing wrinkles. While we have no control over the earth's atmospheric pull, we do, however, have control over the way we direct our skin when we apply our moisturizer or exfoliate; that said, *always* employ the technique of massaging your skin using circular motions or upward and outward shifts—the difference will be worth admiring in the years to come!

- Never stretch or pull the skin under your eyes—this area is very delicate and warrants gentle care. When applying your moisturizer, begin from the inner corner of your eyes and gently pat the tips of your fingers as you move them toward the outer corner of your eyes.

- In choosing your moisturizer, make sure that it contains aloe vera or glycerin as one of its ingredients. Don't worry if it doesn't contain Vitamin E as well—you can always add a few drops of separately bought Vitamin E oil, *or* even prick or cut open a capsule of Vitamin E and add its contents to the dollop of moisturizer that you are about to massage onto your skin.

Fine Lines and Wrinkles

Before you use any of these remedies, make sure that you read the **NOTE** *on Page* 34.

- *Got milk?* It is your biggest anti-wrinkle ally! Before you go to bed each night, soak a cotton pad in cold milk and dab it onto your face and neck. Leave it on until it dries on your skin.

- Cut a few seedless green grapes in half and squeeze out their juice. Soak a cotton pad in this and dab it evenly onto your face and neck. Leave it on for approximately 20 minutes. Employ this remedy as regularly as time permits.

- Mix together 1 teaspoon of plain yogurt and a ¼ teaspoon each of honey, lemon juice, and Vitamin E (*or* sesame) oil. Apply this mixture onto your face and neck. Leave it on for 15–20 minutes.

- To prevent fine lines and wrinkles, especially those that surround your eyes, gently massage your face and neck with a mixture of small, but equal, quantities of honey and glycerin (*or* honey and almond oil) before you go to bed each night. Leave it on overnight. (You can even mix and store either combination of ingredients in a bottle next to your sink—they both make excellent replacements for your bedtime moisturizer.)

FINE LINES AND WRINKLES

- Blend to a smooth pulp ½ a ripe banana (*or* ½ an apple), 1 tablespoon of honey, and 1 egg yolk (optional). Use this facemask once a week for 30–40 minutes to prevent the onset of wrinkles.

- To iron out fine lines, mix 1 teaspoon of carrot juice with 1 tablespoon of honey. Spread this mixture evenly onto your face and neck, and leave it on for 20–25 minutes. Gently cleanse it off using a cotton pad soaked in rosewater, finally rinsing your skin with water.

- Place the white of an egg in a bowl; do not whisk it. Add 1 teaspoon of glycerin (*or* 1 teaspoon of honey) to it, and then gently stir the mixture. Using a cotton pad, evenly smooth this onto your skin, especially covering the fine lines and wrinkles around your eyes and above your lips. Make sure that you do not talk or smile as the egg white begins to dry—this will cause your skin to stretch against the tightening effect of the mask. Leave it on for 30–45 minutes. Soak another cotton pad in rosewater and use it to gently cleanse off the mask, finally rinsing your skin with water. This mask is also effective for the lines on your neck.

- Add a teaspoon of cucumber juice (*or* honey), *or even both,* to *any* of your face and neck masks—among all the other benefits they provide, both of these ingredients possess preventative *and* curative anti-aging properties.

FINE LINES AND WRINKLES

- The natural acids in juices such as pineapple, orange, grape, and tomato, stimulate our skin brilliantly—add a teaspoon of any of these to your face or body masks whenever you concoct them.

- Don't waste your hard-earned money on any expensive anti-wrinkle creams that are corrective due to their enriched content of Vitamin E—you can benefit from the oil without the added cost by buying Vitamin E capsules at any pharmacy instead, (any potency is okay)—prick or cut open 1 capsule each night and mix its contents with your dollop of bedtime moisturizer, or even apply the Vitamin E oil directly onto your skin by itself.

Unwanted Facial Hair

- Mix together small, but equal, quantities of turmeric powder and whole wheat flour. Add just enough sesame oil to form a thick paste. Apply this onto the areas of your face where you'd like to remove any unwanted hair. Leave it on for approximately 30 minutes. Soak your fingertips or a washcloth in lukewarm water and use either to gently exfoliate these areas, finally rinsing your skin with tolerably cold water. (Note: Make sure that you do not over-exfoliate—30 seconds should suffice.) Employ this remedy once a week.

- Mix 2 teaspoons of turmeric powder with just enough milk to form a paste. Apply this evenly onto the areas where you'd like to remove any unwanted facial hair. Leave it on until begins to tighten against your skin, and then rinse it off with tolerably cold water while gently exfoliating your skin. This remedy not only helps to stop the growth of superfluous hair on your face, but also lightens your complexion. (Note: If you find that the turmeric has lent its color to your skin, simply use a cotton pad soaked in milk to cleanse it out.)

- To gradually get rid of any unwanted facial hair, mix together some turmeric powder and just enough warm coconut oil (*or* some gram flour and just enough rosewater) to form a thick paste. Apply either mixture

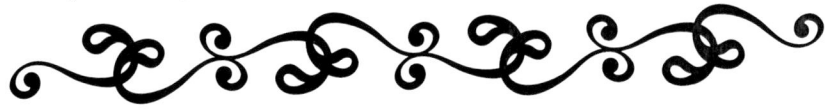

UNWANTED FACIAL HAIR

evenly onto the areas where you'd like to remove any unwanted facial hair. Leave it on for 25–30 minutes. Use your fingertips or a washcloth soaked in lukewarm water to gently exfoliate these areas, finally rinsing your skin with tolerably cold water. (Note: Make sure that you do not over-exfoliate—30 seconds should suffice. Also, if you employ the former remedy and find that the turmeric has lent its color to your skin, simply use a cotton pad soaked in milk to cleanse it out.)

- To weaken and gradually discourage the additional growth of any unwanted facial hair, once a week, *gently* rub a pumice stone in circular motions against the affected areas while you shower. (Note: Make sure that you rub the stone onto these areas *very* gently and for no more than 30 seconds, otherwise you will end up scraping off your skin. Also, do not use this remedy if you have sensitive skin.)

Dry or Chapped Lips

- You might think that licking your lips keeps them moisturized, however, it's quite the opposite, especially in cold weather. As the saliva on your lips evaporates, with it also evaporates your lips' natural moisture. (Since our lips don't have oil glands, their natural moisture is scarce to begin with.) So, instead, always use a lip balm or a chapstick to infuse and sustain moisture—(try picking one that contains honey or Vitamin E as one of its ingredients). Treat your lips to either of these as often as the opportunity presents itself throughout the day, as well as before you go to bed each night. For chapped lips, use a medicated balm or chapstick that contains cooling and soreness-reducing ingredients, such as menthol.

- Gently exfoliate your lips every other day—use a wet, soft toothbrush to gently brush them using circular motions. (You can also use a wet washcloth *or* your bath gloves as effective alternatives while you shower.)

- Replace your matte lipsticks with moisture-rich ones. If you'd rather not waste your existing stock of matte lipsticks, simply make sure that you go over their application on your lips with a tiny bit of lip balm *or* gloss.

Attain a Smooth and Radiant Complexion

Before you use any of these remedies, make sure that you read the **NOTE** *on Page* 34.

- Blend to a smooth pulp ½ a ripe banana and 4 tablespoons of cold milk. Apply this pack onto your face and neck for approximately 20 minutes.

- Mix 4–5 drops of lemon juice with 2 teaspoons of gram flour and just enough milk to form a thick paste. Apply this mixture onto your face and neck for approximately 15 minutes.

- Make a paste by mixing together a ¼ teaspoon each of turmeric and sandalwood powders, 1½ tablespoons of clotted cream, and 1 tablespoon of gram flour. Apply this evenly onto your face and neck, and leave it on for approximately 30 minutes. Employ this remedy once a week.

- Using a mini blender, puree together 1 unpeeled, raw carrot and 1 teaspoon each of orange juice and olive (*or* almond) oil. Apply this mixture onto your face and neck, and leave it on for 5–7 minutes.

- Mix 2 tablespoons of freshly pureed tomato with 1 teaspoon of lemon juice and a ¼ teaspoon of glycerin. Apply this onto your skin and leave it on for approximately 25 minutes.

ATTAIN A SMOOTH AND RADIANT COMPLEXION

- Crush a teaspoon's worth of fresh basil leaves (*or* a teaspoon's worth of fresh mint leaves); then add to this paste 1 tablespoon of honey and 4–5 drops of lemon juice. Apply this mixture onto your face and neck. Leave it on for approximately 20 minutes. This remedy is also effective when used to reduce the appearance of blemishes on your skin.

- Don't have much time to concoct a mask? Use a cotton pad to dab some cold orange juice onto your face and neck; leave it on until it dries.

- Add honey to *any* of your facial masks, or, if nothing else, use honey as a mask by itself.

- Don't waste your precious money on any expensive exfoliating products that claim to be "magical" for your skin, such as rotating brushes or creams with microbeads—a wet washcloth (*or* a pair of exfoliating bath gloves *or* a loofah) does *just as good a job* in giving you the same exfoliating benefits—use any one of these two-to-three times a week when you shower, also gently exfoliating your face and neck with it. (Note: Never over-exfoliate! You will end up sloughing off not only the dead cells on the surface of your skin, but also the healthy ones underneath that protect you from damaging factors like the sun's rays or pollution.)

NECK

If you have watched infomercials that promote expensive, anti-aging products or gadgets that all promise to take five-to-ten years off your age, then you've probably observed that these ads typically sport mature models who indulge us in *before* and *after* close-up shots, so that we can examine the differences in their appearance. While their freshly brushed faces indeed seem to look restored and radiant, if you've taken notice of the skin on their necks, it usually appears to tell a different story.

In caring for our skin, we seem to be overly conscious and corrective about our facial skin. What most fail to recognize is that our neck is *also* an extension of our face, and without proper care, it is just as susceptible to lines and sagging skin, both of which take away from our appearance.

It is never too late to start giving this commonly neglected part of your body the attention it deserves, so that it can begin to look just as pampered as your face.

- To reduce the appearance of any lines on your neck, place the white of an egg in a bowl; do not whisk it. Add 1 teaspoon of glycerin (*or* 1 teaspoon

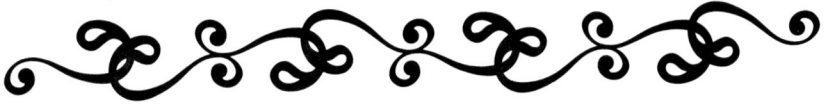

of honey) to it, and then gently stir the mixture. Using a cotton pad, evenly smooth this onto the affected areas of your skin. Leave it on for 30–45 minutes. Soak another cotton pad in rosewater and use it to gently cleanse off the mask, finally rinsing your skin with tolerably cold water. This mask is also effective for the fine lines and wrinkles around your eyes and above your lips, but if you also use it on those areas, make sure that you do not talk or smile as the egg white begins to dry—this will cause your skin to stretch against the tightening effect of the mask.

- Another remedy for the lines on your neck is to mix 1 tablespoon of gram flour with just enough lemon juice to form a paste. Apply this evenly onto your skin and leave it on until it begins to dry. Rinse it off with tolerably cold water. This remedy is also effective for treating over-pigmented elbows and knees.

- Stay away from peel-off masks—they pull and stretch your delicate skin when they're taken off. Instead, exfoliate your skin using a wet washcloth *or* a pair of coarse bath gloves in the shower.

- Whenever you moisturize or exfoliate your face, *always* extend the treatment to your neck. In doing so, use upward motions at all times. Also, each time you employ a remedy that involves the application of a facemask, always apply the concoction to *both* your face and neck. In implementing these beauty do's, don't forget to lavish the back of your neck as well!

ARMS, TORSO, AND LEGS

You've probably heard this over and over again, but it is, nonetheless, *very* worthy of repetition—the sun *is* one of our skin's biggest enemies in disguise—don't let its deceivingly inviting warmth lure you into sun-bathing. The bronzed look that you strive so hard to attain will have come at the price of your skin's exposure to dangerously harmful ultraviolet (UV) rays. The damage caused by these rays is collective, and your skin will blatantly reveal this fact year after year, leaving you vulnerably exposed to consequences that may bare themselves in the form of premature aging, various skin disorders, *and more*. So protect yourself from any unnecessary exposure to the sun, and try to incorporate the following basics into your day:

- ❋ Don't leave your home without a sunscreen *or* sunblock lotion that contains a Sun Protection Factor (SPF) of *at least* 15 or more. (Note, however, that higher the SPF, longer the protection.)
- ❋ Over and above limiting your time in the sun, try to avoid its direct rays between the hours of 11:00 a.m. and 3:00 p.m.
- ❋ Wear clothing that protects your skin.

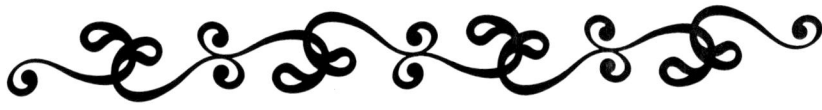

ARMS, TORSO, AND LEGS

Remember that the skin on your body contributes to your overall image, and therefore, needs to be in harmony with the skin on your face and neck. The remedies in this section will help you to not only indulge your skin, but also repair some of the damage it might have endured due to lack of care or over-exposure to the sun.

- Pamper yourself once a week by soaking in a bath. 10–15 minutes before you bathe, massage some coconut oil onto your body. Your skin will become supple and luminous.

- Pour 1 cup of milk (*or* 1 cup of apple juice) in your bath water—either of these will leave your skin feeling baby-soft.

- If you have dry skin, before you go to bed each night, massage onto it a mixture made from 2 parts of Vitamin E oil and 1 part of glycerin, making sure that you concoct just the quantity that your skin will easily absorb. Employ this remedy for about a week, or longer, if needed.

- For over-pigmented elbows and knees, cut a lemon in half and sprinkle onto it some coarse sugar granules. Using circular motions, gently scrub the affected areas with it for approximately 2 minutes each, lightly squeezing some juice out of the lemon from time-to-time.

- Another remedy for dark elbows and knees is to mix 1 tablespoon of gram flour with just enough lemon juice to form a paste. Apply this mixture onto the affected areas and leave it on until it begins to dry. Rinse it off in the shower, or cleanse your skin using a wet washcloth. This remedy is also effectively used to reduce the appearance of any lines on your neck.

- If you have dry elbows and knees, mash up some pineapple, (fresh is ideal, but canned will work too). Rub the pulp onto the affected areas. Leave it on for approximately 15 minutes before you rinse it off. Massage on a few drops of almond oil, followed by a thin top layer of glycerin. (If you don't have 15 minutes to spare, use a slice of pineapple as you would a sponge or a loofah to scrub the affected areas in the shower.)

- If you have scars or blemishes on your body, mix together equal quantities of honey and orange juice. Using a cotton pad, apply this mixture onto the affected areas, and leave it on for approximately 10 minutes before you rinse it off in the shower.

- Another remedy to reduce the appearance of scars or blemishes is to mix together equal quantities each of cucumber juice (*or* glycerin), lemon juice, and rosewater. If possible, cleanse the affected areas with a wet

ARMS, TORSO, AND LEGS

washcloth before you apply this mixture. Leave it on for approximately 45 minutes. Employ this remedy as regularly as time permits—it will not only clarify your skin, but also help it stay that way. This remedy can also be effectively used on your face to treat pimples, acne, and blemishes.

- Repair blemished skin by crushing a teaspoon's worth of fresh basil leaves (*or* a teaspoon's worth of fresh mint leaves) and then adding to this paste 1 tablespoon of honey and 4–5 drops of lemon juice. Apply this mixture onto the affected areas of your skin and leave it on for approximately 20 minutes. Rinse it off in the shower, or cleanse it using a wet washcloth. This remedy not only reduces the appearance of blemishes, but also lends your skin a healthy glow.

- To attain radiant skin, blend to a smooth pulp some papaya and three times the quantity of aloe vera oil. Apply this mixture onto your skin for *no more than* 5–10 minutes before you shower, making sure that you avoid sensitive areas. Employ this remedy once a month.

- To relieve the stinging sensation caused by sunburn, use a cotton pad to lightly dab the affected areas with apple cider vinegar. When it dries up, dab on a second coat and allow it to dry as well. Rinse your skin in the shower with tolerably cool water.

ARMS, TORSO, AND LEGS

- Another remedy to relieve the pain caused by sunburn is to mix the white of an egg with approximately the same quantity of glycerin. Using a cotton pad, smooth this mixture onto the affected areas of your skin and leave it on for 20–25 minutes. Rinse it off in the shower using tolerably cool water.

- To soothe skin inflammation or the swelling that results from sunburn, puree ½ a cucumber in a mini blender and apply this onto the affected areas. Leave it on for approximately 20 minutes before rinsing it off with tolerably cool water.

- If you have stretch marks on your body, use circular motions to massage onto the affected areas some olive (*or* Vitamin E) oil. Do this for 15–20 minutes before you go to bed each night, making sure that you leave the application on overnight. (Note: Once you develop stretch marks, unfortunately, you cannot completely eliminate them; however, you can reduce their appearance. If you are pregnant, you can employ this remedy to *prevent* their occurrence in the first place.)

- If you are struggling with stubborn cellulite, while you shower, use upward strokes to massage the affected areas with a bristled brush, *or* a loofah, *or* a pair of exfoliating bath gloves. Employ this remedy once a week for 5–10 minutes (or less, if you have sensitive skin). Like stretch marks, you

ARMS, TORSO, AND LEGS

cannot completely get rid of cellulite, but you can definitely improve its appearance by inducing your blood circulation to the affected areas.

- Moisturize your skin *everyday,* no exceptions! It is one of the most important and rewarding steps that you can implement in your beauty routine. Use moisturizers that contain aloe vera *or* glycerin as one of their ingredients. Do not worry if they don't contain Vitamin E as well—you can always add a few drops of separately bought Vitamin E oil, *or* even prick or cut open a capsule of Vitamin E and add its contents to the dollop of moisturizer that you are about to massage onto your skin. Also, treat your hands to a small amount of moisturizer several times a day, especially after you've washed them—it'll keep them supple.

- Use a washcloth, *or* a loofah, *or* a pair of coarse bath gloves in the shower—each of these effectively exfoliates your skin by sloughing off any dead cells on its surface, thereby exposing the satin-smooth skin underneath. The process of exfoliating also stimulates your blood circulation in those areas. (Note: To delay the effects of gravity, always scrub your skin in the upward direction.)

NAILS

Although they form a small a part of our bodies, our nails are nonetheless very significant—they help protect the sensitive and nerve-rich tips of our fingers and toes from injury. Abnormalities in them can surface in various forms, such as discoloration, horizontal or vertical ridges, dryness, or brittleness—these may often be a sign of an ongoing internal health problem or external injury. However, irregularities in our nails can also result from the lack of proper care or hygiene. It is therefore very important for us to keep our nails groomed. Manicures and pedicures help us achieve just that—they are not purely cosmetic, they also promote healthy nails—their processes involve sloughing off dead skin on and around our nails, as well as a gentle massage on our hands and feet, which, in turn, promotes the circulation of blood to those areas. (Note: If you go to a salon for these services, be aware that shared nail tools and footbaths have the potential to transmit fungal or bacterial infections.)

The tips in this section will help you with some of the most common problems that we encounter with our nails.

NAILS

- Protect your nails from becoming brittle by shielding them from elements such as harsh soaps or detergents, chemicals, and cold weather. Wearing a pair of gloves not only prevents their exposure to such elements, but also helps them retain their moisture.

- Refrain from using acetone-based polish removers. They contain chemicals that rob your nails of moisture, causing them to chip and break easily.

- Strengthen brittle nails by smearing onto them some olive oil (*or* a mixture of a few drops each of honey and almond oil) before you go to bed each night. (Note: Make sure that you put on a pair of gloves to hold the moisture to your nails and also protect your sheets.)

- Always soak your nails in lukewarm water for *at least* 10 minutes before you trim them—doing so makes them soft, flexible, and easier to cut; it also makes them more resistant to chipping while they're being trimmed. (This remedy is especially helpful if you suffer from ingrown toenails.)

- Buff your nails each time you give yourself a manicure or pedicure. Doing so evens out the surface of your nails *and* increases the blood circulation to them.

NAILS

- One of the main causes of yellow nails is darker shades of polish. A simple and inexpensive way to bleach out the yellow from your nails is to use a small wedge of fresh lemon—rub this against each fingernail as if you were using it to remove your nail polish.

- From time-to-time, give your nails a rest from polish. Nail polish dries out our nails, making them susceptible to breakage. When you do wear polish, make sure that you use a strengthening basecoat to protect your nails.

- Steer clear of uncomfortably tight footwear *or* dirty socks—both of these can cause you toenail infections.

- *Whenever* you moisturize your hands or feet, remember to extend the luxury to your nails as well.

FEET

Our feet are our hardest-working body parts, and yet, also one of our most neglected. Lack of proper care for them bares itself in various forms—corns, blisters, calluses, and cracked skin, to name a few. Regardless of how healthy your hair and skin might be, if you feature a pair of feet that are in bad need of some attention, they will, without doubt, qualify as a show-stopper.

That said, use the remedies in this section to give your feet the attention that they have rightfully earned. (Note: Make sure that you put on a pair of socks to hold any application to your skin and also protect your floors and sheets.)

- If you are fighting a losing battle with dry skin on your feet, before you go to bed each night, wash and dry them well, and then massage onto them a small amount of warm olive, sesame, coconut, *or* almond oil—each of these oils make an *excellent* conditioner for your skin. You can even use a few drops of either oil after a pedicure, instead of your normal moisturizer. This remedy also works effectively if you suffer from cracked skin on your soles.

- If the skin on your soles is split or fissured, form a thick paste by mixing 1 tablespoon of sandalwood powder with equal quantities each of mustard

FEET

and coconut oils—apply this mixture onto the affected areas before you go to bed each night.

- Another remedy for split or fissured skin on your soles is to mix 1 teaspoon of turmeric powder with just enough castor oil to form a thick paste. Before you shower, apply this onto the affected areas and leave it on for 15–20 minutes. (Note: In using this remedy, make sure that you put on *two* pairs of socks to protect your floors—turmeric stains are difficult to wash out!)

- If you suffer from hardened or cracked skin on your heels, *at least* once a week, before you go to bed, mix 4 tablespoons of kitchen salt in some warm water. Soak your feet in this mixture for 10–15 minutes—this will help soften the rough and scaly skin on your soles, making it easier to slough off. Use a pumice stone *or* a callus remover to gently scrub the affected areas. (Note: Make sure that you do not scrub too hard—the goal is to simply get rid of a few layers of dead skin each time you use this remedy, gradually working your way toward soft and supple feet.) Rinse your feet in the same salt water, and then dry them well before massaging on a mixture of a few drops each of castor oil and lemon juice. Follow this routine until you are satisfied with the results.

- If your feet are tired and painful, soak them for 10–15 minutes in a footbath made from some warm water, ½ a cup of rosewater, and 4 tablespoons of kitchen salt.

FEET

- To attain soft and supple skin on your feet, massage onto them a small amount of glycerin before you go to bed each night.

- If you suffer from foot perspiration, dust your feet with sandalwood powder each day—it has tremendous cooling properties and is naturally fragrant.

- If the shoe doesn't fit…don't wear it! Tight shoes compress your skin, thereby encouraging the formation of corns and calluses. Furthermore, they interfere with the circulation of blood, causing other foot-related problems.

- The next time you give yourself a pedicure, add a dollop of shampoo to your foot soak—you will find your soles easier to scrub; also, the presence of shampoo in your foot soak will improve the texture of your toenails, making them easier to groom.

- For calluses on your soles, keep a pumice stone *or* a callus remover in your shower, so that you can conveniently give the affected areas a quick scrub each day. After your shower, apply onto your feet a small amount of moisturizer *or* oil.

- *Whenever* you moisturize your body as part of your daily routine, also remember to treat your feet!

MAKE YOUR OWN BEAUTY ESSENTIALS

One of the most luxurious and comprehensive care routines for our skin is none other than a facial. Many indulge in this treatment without knowing the extent to which it is beneficial for our skin. This section first outlines the steps that are involved in a facial, and then gives you sample recipes that you can use to concoct your own cleansers, astringents, toners, and facemasks.

Facials typically involve (in this order):

* a cleansing procedure (which also includes the brief use of an exfoliant);
* a face and neck massage;
* facial steaming; and
* a facemask application.

Each one of these steps plays an important role and yields several different benefits. The cleansing procedure removes any impurities on our skin. The use of an exfoliant during this step helps to slough off any dead cells on the surface of our skin, exposing a fresh and soft layer of skin underneath. A face and neck massage helps to improve our blood circulation in those areas.

This, in turn, stimulates the release of toxins that are embedded beneath our skin. This step also doubles up in relaxing our facial muscles, enabling a delay in the onset of wrinkles. Facial steaming opens up our pores, making it easy to deep-clean any dirt and oil deposits in them. Open pores further allow our skin to better absorb the subsequent facemask. Steaming also helps to soften blackheads and whiteheads, so that they can be extracted easily. Finally, the application of a facemask at the tail end of the process helps to tone, moisturize, and replenish our skin.

Cleansers, Astringents, and Toners

- Watermelon juice makes a very refreshing cleanser. Using a fork, mash a small piece of this fruit. Soak a cotton pad in its juice and gently dab it onto your skin. Rinse it off after approximately 5 minutes.

- Before you go to bed each night, cleanse your skin with either almond, olive, *or* sesame oil. Massage any one of these generously onto your face and neck. Soak a washcloth in lukewarm water, wring it out, and then use it to gently wipe the oil off your skin. (Each of these oils also effectively cleanses makeup, even if the makeup is waterproof.)

- Mix the juice of ½ a lemon and ½ an orange with 6 tablespoons of rosewater. Using a fine strainer, filter out the resulting astringent. Use a cotton pad to cleanse your skin with it. (You can either bottle and refrigerate this astringent for daily use, or adjust the quantities of the ingredients as needed for fewer applications, in the proportions listed above.)

- Lemon juice is a potent astringent. Dilute it with some rosewater, and then use it to cleanse your skin. You will experience a little tingling sensation as it dries, but it will leave your skin feeling highly refreshed. (Note: Be careful to keep this mixture from entering your eyes. Also, if you have dry skin, use a combination of more rosewater and less lemon juice.)

CLEANSERS, ASTRINGENTS, AND TONERS

- Mix together 1 tablespoon each of cucumber juice and lemon juice. Add to this a ¼ teaspoon of turmeric powder. Using a cotton pad, gently cleanse your skin with the resulting astringent, evenly dabbing the remaining mixture onto your face and neck. Leave it on until it begins to dry, and then rinse it off with tolerably cold water. This astringent not only cleanses your skin, but also lightens your complexion.

- Blend together ½ an unpeeled cucumber, 6 teaspoons of rosewater, and 3 teaspoons of glycerin. Using a fine strainer, filter out the resulting toner. Use a cotton pad to dab it onto your face and neck. Leave it on for approximately 15 minutes, and then rinse it off with tolerably cold water. (You can either bottle and refrigerate this toner for daily use on your face and body, or adjust the quantities of the ingredients as needed for fewer applications, in the proportions listed above.)

- Cut a tomato in half. Using circular motions, gently scrub your face and neck with its insides. This remedy not only tones and refines your pores, but also lightens your complexion.

- To tighten your pores, use a cotton pad to evenly smooth a whisked egg white onto your skin. Leave it on for approximately 15 minutes, and then rinse it off with tolerably cold water.

CLEANSERS, ASTRINGENTS, AND TONERS

- A great skin toner is none other than an ice-cube. Glide an ice-cube or two against your skin to tighten your pores *and* increase your blood circulation to those areas. (If you have an ice-cube tray at home, ice-cubes made using rosewater are even more effective as skin toners—in addition to benefiting you as described above, they leave your skin feeling petal-soft.)

Natural Exfoliants

Note: In using exfoliants on your skin, make sure that you never over-exfoliate—(30 seconds is usually adequate)—otherwise, you will end up sloughing off not only the dead cells on the surface of your skin, but also the healthy ones underneath that protect you from damaging factors like the sun's rays or pollution.

- Blend together 2–3 small strawberries and 1 teaspoon of clotted cream. Gently scrub your face and neck with this mixture.

- Exfoliate your skin with a scrub made from ½ a teaspoon each of glycerin and lemon juice, 1 teaspoon of olive oil, and 1 tablespoon of coarse sugar granules.

- Gently scrub your face and neck with a mixture made from equal quantities of kitchen salt and almond oil.

- Mix 1 teaspoon each of almond powder, desiccated coconut, and rosewater with 1½ teaspoons of mashed, plain yogurt. Apply this mask evenly onto your face and neck. Leave it on for 20–25 minutes. Soak the tips of your fingers in cold water (*or* milk) and begin to gently exfoliate your skin while scrubbing off the mask. (Note: Use circular motions on your face and upward strokes on your neck.)

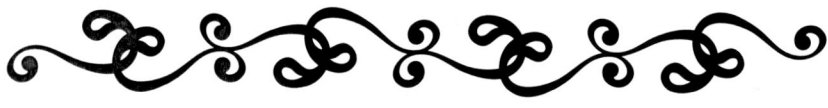

- Try this out-of-the-ordinary scrub—soak 2 tablespoons of whole green lentils overnight. In the morning, rinse them two-to-three times before grinding them coarsely. Stir in 1 tablespoon each of honey and coconut oil. Apply this mixture evenly onto your face and neck. Leave it on for 10–15 minutes, and then begin to gently exfoliate your skin while scrubbing off the pack.

Facemasks

There is no hard and fast rule when it comes to the concoction of facemasks using natural ingredients—you can be as creative as your kitchen will let you be! The concoctions in this section have been presented as examples to show you how much versatility *every single* ingredient affords you. So, no matter what combination of ingredients you use, whether based on availability, allergy, or even pure choice, you will find much comfort in the fact that each ingredient is free of the chemicals and preservatives found in commercial beauty products. That said, have fun with the ingredients and pick what fancies you on a given day, or look up the benefits of specific ingredients in the section, "**ABOUT THE INGREDIENTS**," and customize a concoction to suit your needs!

Before you begin, do take note of the following tips—they will enable you to get the most out of your facemask:

* Always apply your concoction of choice to *both* your face and neck, preferably after you have cleansed your skin;

* Leave your facemask application on for *at least* 25 minutes, unless it begins to dry and tighten on your skin sooner;

* Always use tolerably cold water to rinse it off, unless you used any oil as an ingredient in it, in which case, you should use lukewarm water for your final rinse—cold water tightens your pores, sealing in the nourishment from the

FACEMASKS

ingredients that you used, whereas lukewarm water works best to gently dissolve and cleanse any excess oil left on your skin after a facemask;

- ✲ If you have the time, glide an ice-cube or two against your skin, preferably one that is made from rosewater;
- ✲ Finally, apply a few drops of moisturizer *or* oil (almond, olive, *or* Vitamin E) onto your skin.

You can also extend the luxury of your facemasks to your body—note that the ingredient quantities suggested for each concoction in this section should suffice for an application on your face and neck; adjust them proportionately, if you plan to use that application on your body. Also, to thicken the texture of any facemask, feel free to add ingredients such as an egg yoke, plain yogurt, honey, *or* gram flour. Get creative!

- Whisk together 1 teaspoon each of honey and plain yogurt, 2 teaspoons of lemon juice, and 1 egg white.

- Mix 1 tablespoon of gram flour with a ¼ teaspoon of sandalwood powder, ½ a teaspoon each of honey and clotted cream, and just enough rosewater to form a paste.

- Blend to a smooth pulp ½ a ripe banana and 1 teaspoon each of milk, rosewater, and almond oil.

FACEMASKS

- Blend 1 teaspoon's worth each of pineapple and papaya with 2 teaspoons of honey. Apply this mask and leave it on for *no more than* 5–10 minutes.

- Mix 1 teaspoon of lemon juice with ½ a teaspoon of glycerin and 2 teaspoons of rosewater.

- Puree together ½ a tablespoon of plain yogurt, 1 teaspoon's worth of an unpeeled cucumber, 1 small strawberry, and ½ a teaspoon of honey.

- Mix together 1 teaspoon each of honey, lemon juice, orange juice, and plain yogurt.

- In a bowl, whisk 1 egg with 1 teaspoon each of coconut oil and honey.

- Use a mini blender to puree together ½ a tablespoon of milk, 1 teaspoon's worth of an unpeeled cucumber, and ½ a teaspoon each of plain yogurt and sandalwood powder.

- Blend together 1 egg white, 4 seedless green grapes, and ½ a teaspoon each of lemon juice and almond oil.

- In a bowl, whisk together 1 egg yolk, 1 teaspoon of honey, and a ¼ teaspoon each of Vitamin E and almond oils.

FACEMASKS

- Using a mini blender, puree together 1 tablespoon's worth of your choice of fruit, and ½ a tablespoon each of clotted cream and gram flour.

- Mix together 1 egg white, 1 teaspoon of honey, ½ a teaspoon of glycerin, and just enough gram flour to form a paste.

- Mix together 1 tablespoon each of honey and plain yogurt (*or* milk).

- Using a mini blender, puree together ½ a teaspoon of plain yogurt, 1½ teaspoons of gram flour, and 1 teaspoon's worth each of a tomato and an unpeeled cucumber.

- Whisk together 1 egg yolk, ½ a teaspoon each of plain yogurt, lemon juice, rosewater, and apple juice, and 3–4 drops each of glycerin and almond oil.

- If you're extremely sparse on time, you can *never* go wrong with a plain honey mask!

ABOUT THE INGREDIENTS

Natural beauty home remedies are not, by any means, a new-age discovery—they've been used for centuries around the world. Interestingly, the benefits of natural ingredients were discovered purely out of necessity, based on trial-and-error. The healing powers demonstrated by these ingredients over the generations that followed, rightfully earned them their privilege to be used for remedial purposes.

While there are several books and websites that recommend natural ingredients in their beauty remedies, many use painfully complex words to describe the therapeutic benefits of each ingredient—for example, anti-phlogistic, cicatrisant, emollient, or vulnerary—which are non-comprehensible and also intimidating to a vast majority of us using those remedies. This section alphabetically lists all the ingredients suggested in this book and further outlines, in uncomplicated terms, how each ingredient plays an important role in any remedy for which it is used.

A Reminder about the Ingredients: Do not use *any* ingredient referenced herein if you are aware of any sensitivity or allergy that you may have to that

ingredient. Consult a licensed healthcare provider (and also test a small area of your skin well in advance) if you are unsure about using an ingredient.

Almond Oil or Powder

Almonds contain silica, a vital mineral used by our bodies to maintain the healthy growth of skin, hair, and nails. Used in either form, they have proven themselves to be hydrating and nourishing for both our skin and hair. Used on skin, almonds improve our complexion by fighting dry skin, dark circles, uneven pigmentation, and blackheads. Almond oil is easily absorbed by our pores—its regular use makes our skin soft and supple, preventing *and* reducing the appearance of fine lines and wrinkles. Furthermore, due to its ability to infuse moisture, this ingredient is effectively used in remedies to treat brittle nails and help us attain a smooth and radiant complexion. Used on hair, almond oil successfully combats a multitude of hair and scalp-related problems, such as dull or dry hair, breakage and split ends, premature graying, dandruff, and hair loss.

Aloe Vera Oil or Juice

Very widely used in beauty products, aloe vera is known for its ability to rebuild our skin. It possesses anti-inflammatory properties that aid in healing pimples, acne, skin wounds, and sunburn, *all* with reduced scarring.

Furthermore, due to its tremendous ability to infuse moisture, aloe vera is also successfully used in remedies to treat dry skin *and* prevent the formation of fine lines and wrinkles.

Apples or Apple Juice

Apples contain silica, a vital mineral used by our bodies to maintain the healthy growth of skin, hair, and nails. Used in either form, this fruit acts as a *very* nutritional toner and conditioner for our skin, leaving skin soft and supple; this, in turn, enables it to be effectively used in remedies to delay the onset of wrinkles. Furthermore, apples possess the ability to soak up any excess oil on the surface of our skin; they work relentlessly to combat occurrences of pimples, acne, and blemishes. They've been used as a natural remedy for centuries because of these very healing powers.

Bananas

Although their presence in beauty products is not as common as that of other fruits, bananas make a rich conditioner for our skin. Besides fighting dryness and the onset of fine lines and wrinkles, they aid in restoring the radiance in our skin. They are also used in remedies to clear troubled skin of pimples and acne, helping it regain a soft and supple texture. When used on hair, bananas effectively demonstrate their restorative attributes, especially on dry or damaged hair.

ABOUT THE INGREDIENTS

Basil Leaves (Fresh)

Primarily known for its culinary uses, basil has been found to also possess extraordinary healing powers, when applied externally. This ingredient has the ability to stimulate the circulation of blood, and therefore aids in reviving dull skin and further restoring its radiance. Used with other ingredients, basil leaves also reduce, if not eliminate, blemishes, dark circles, and instances of uneven pigmentation. Their juice makes an effective cleanser and toner for our skin, (*including* that on our scalp)—it is therefore used in remedies to successfully combat pimples and acne, as well as oily hair.

Black Pepper

Black pepper is known to have significant antioxidant and antibacterial properties. It is also a powerful stimulant and promotes the circulation of blood. When used with other ingredients on hair, it aids in slowing down the process of premature graying. It does so by stimulating the production of a pigment called melanin in our hair follicles, the tiny sacs under our skin in which our hair is formed. (This pigment is the primary determinant of hair and skin color, and the presence of increased amounts of melanin in our follicles, translates to darker hair color. Conversely, when our bodies reduce or stop the production of this pigment, our hair becomes colorless, a term more commonly known as gray hair.)

ABOUT THE INGREDIENTS

Buttermilk

Characterized by its tartness, cultured buttermilk contains a rich amount of lactic acid, which is a pure indulgence for dry or depleted skin. Used with lemon juice to reduce the appearance of freckles, buttermilk plays a complementary role by cooling and moisturizing our skin, while the lemon juice acts as a potent astringent and bleaching agent.

Carrots or Carrot Juice

Due to their rich Vitamin A content, carrots possess the ability to make our skin glow. Like cucumbers and potatoes, the benefits of carrots lie in their skin—they are the most effective when used unpeeled. Carrot juice is an excellent toner for oily skin and aids in fighting off pimples and blemishes. It is also used in remedies to successfully treat fine lines and forming wrinkles. (Note: Carrots may stain your skin if left on for too long—when using them as the main ingredient in your masks, make sure that you leave the mixture on for no more than 10 minutes. If you find that your skin has nonetheless absorbed some color, simply use a cotton pad soaked in milk to cleanse it out.)

Castor Oil

Castor oil is extremely versatile in its use. It possesses the remarkable ability to penetrate our skin and hair deeply, and is therefore employed in a

multitude of remedies to restore the luster to dull or dry hair, reduce hair loss *and also* stimulate hair growth on not only our scalp, but also our eyebrows and eyelashes. Furthermore, this oil is known to work wonders when used to soothe and repair our skin—it is *just as* effective on the delicate skin around our eyes, as it is on the tough skin on the soles of our feet—it is therefore successfully employed in remedies to treat tired and puffy eyes, as well as any cracked or hardened skin on our soles.

Cinnamon Powder

A spice popular for its ability to tingle our senses thorough its aroma, cinnamon may very well be known primarily for its culinary uses, however, this spice is very versatile and can also be used externally. It possesses tremendous antibacterial properties—when applied onto our skin, it acts as an antiseptic astringent, making it very effective in remedies to cure pimples and acne. Cinnamon powder is also a strong stimulant—it unfailingly promotes the circulation of blood. For this reason, it is known to aid in reversing hair loss when applied onto our scalp.

Clotted Cream

Clotted cream is a thick, yellow cream which forms when unpasteurized whole milk is boiled and then left to cool in shallow pans for several hours, causing its cream content to rise to the surface and clot. It contains approximately 55% of

butter fat. Commonly known as *Malai* in India and *Clotted* or *Devonshire* cream in the West, this ingredient makes an excellent skin moisturizer—in fact, it has proven itself as an effective winter-skincare solution. Its use in remedies never fails to help us attain a smooth, supple, and radiant complexion. Furthermore, clotted cream is also known for its ability to reduce the appearance of dark circles and correct any instances of uneven pigmentation.

Coconut Oil or Milk

Used in either form, this fruit makes an *immensely* nourishing conditioner for both our skin and hair. Although it is extremely gentle, it possesses the ability to infuse moisture and penetrate even the tough skin on the soles of our feet—it has therefore found use in remedies to treat cracked or hardened skin on our soles. Its moisturizing attribute further allows coconut oil to be successfully used in remedies to restore the radiance in a dull complexion, as well as treat dry skin, fine lines and wrinkles, *and* dark circles. Used on hair, it combats problems such as dull or dry hair, dandruff, hair loss, and premature graying.

Cucumbers

Used in several beauty products on the market today, cucumbers are rightfully recognized as a *food for our skin*—they contain elements that help our skin maintain its elasticity, further preventing the onset of fine lines and wrinkles. Due to their undoubted ability to moisturize and repair our skin, they have

found use in a multitude of remedies to treat dry skin, reduce the appearance of freckles or blemishes, heal sun-damaged skin, as well as restore the radiance to a dark or dull complexion. Cucumber juice also has a very cooling effect on our skin; when applied, it tightens our pores, acting as an effective, yet gentle, toner. On the other hand, it possesses mild astringent properties that qualify it as an excellent cleanser as well. These two attributes enable it to be successfully used in remedies to treat oily skin, which, in turn, prevents the occurrence of pimples and acne. The use of cucumbers in remedies also helps to soothe tired eyes, reduce the puffiness around eyes, and rectify dark circles. Like carrots and potatoes, the benefits of cucumbers lie in their skin—they are the most effective when used unpeeled.

Cumin Powder

Cumin powder is commonly known for its culinary uses. Applied externally, however, it makes an effective remedy for pimples, acne, and blemishes due to its rich content of thymol, a substance that possesses antiseptic properties.

Curry Leaves

Highly aromatic, this ingredient is known to many for its extensive use in Indian cuisine. However, it has also proven its effectiveness in preventing premature graying—curry leaves possess remarkable properties that restore the vitality in our hair follicles, the tiny sacs under our skin in which our hair

is formed, enabling them to stimulate their production of a pigment called melanin. (This pigment is the primary determinant of hair and skin color, and the presence of increased amounts of melanin in our follicles, translates to darker hair color. Conversely, when our bodies reduce or stop the production of this pigment, our hair becomes colorless, a term more commonly known as gray hair.) While fresh curry leaves have a short shelf life, you can preserve them for a longer period by storing them in your freezer.

Desiccated Coconut

Desiccated coconut is none other than dehydrated and shredded white coconut meat. It is primarily known for its culinary uses; however, its coarse texture also makes it a very effective exfoliant—when used for this purpose, desiccated coconut gently sloughs off any dead cells on the surface of our skin, while yet immensely nourishing and conditioning it.

Eggs

Eggs contain Vitamin E and other antioxidants, which are very essential for healthy skin and hair. Both the egg white and the yolk provide our skin and hair with nourishment. Egg whites are known to tighten pores, and are therefore regarded as a good skin toner, *especially* if you have oily skin; this, in turn, helps them prevent clogged pores and the subsequent formation of blackheads. Furthermore, the ability of egg whites to tighten our pores

enables them to aid in treating oily hair, reducing the puffiness around our eyes, and minimizing the appearance of lines on our neck. One of the proteins contained in them also possesses antiseptic properties, making egg whites effective in remedies for pimples, acne, blemishes, and sunburn. Egg yolks, on the other hand, are a potent conditioner—they contain a substance known as lecithin, which lends our skin and hair moisture and radiance; they are therefore used to enrich facemasks and shampoos. They are very versatile and have found use in a multitude of remedies to effectively treat dry skin, fine lines and wrinkles, dull or dry hair, dandruff, and hair loss.

Eggplant

The eggplant contains antioxidants, the presence of which makes it effective as an aid when used in remedies to reduce the appearance of freckles.

Fuller's Earth

Rich in minerals, fuller's earth is known for its ability to absorb impurities from our skin. Due to this attribute, it makes an excellent deep-cleansing remedy for oily skin. Used with other ingredients to form clay masks, it effectively combats pimples, acne, and blemishes. Furthermore, similar to sandalwood powder, fuller's earth is *very* cooling for our skin; its use in remedies not only treats sunburn, but also reduces the appearance of freckles, which are triggered by exposure to the sun. (Note: Use *only* the cosmetic

grade of fuller's earth, which is commonly classified on its label using terms such as "100% Pure," "Sterilized," and "High Quality Fine Grade Powder.")

Glycerin

Glycerin is a humectant—it attracts moisture to our skin, and then helps our skin to retain that moisture, leaving it feeling soft and supple. It is a gentle and skin-loving ingredient. For these very reasons, it is used as a base in many commercial lotions and creams—it successfully treats dry skin, restores the radiance to a dull complexion, relieves the pain caused by sunburn, prevents premature aging, and even minimizes the appearance of fine lines, wrinkles, and lines on our neck. Used on hair, it effectively restores the luster in dull or dry hair.

Gooseberry Oil or Powder

Extremely rich in Vitamin C, gooseberry makes a *very* effective hair tonic. It is used in remedies to cure a multitude of hair and scalp-related problems, such as dull or dry hair, dandruff, and hair loss. Furthermore, its use strengthens our strands and promotes hair growth. This sour fruit also makes an excellent remedy for premature graying—it possesses the ability to stimulate the production of a pigment called melanin in our hair follicles, the tiny sacs under our skin in which our hair is formed. (This pigment is the primary determinant of hair and skin color, and the presence of increased amounts of melanin in our follicles, translates to darker hair color. Conversely, when

our bodies reduce or stop the production of this pigment, our hair becomes colorless, a term more commonly known as gray hair.)

Gram Flour

Commonly referred to as chickpeas *or* garbanzo beans, grams contain a high amount of protein. Their flour is very versatile in nature and is used in remedies for both our skin and hair. Used on skin, gram flour aids in reversing a dry or dull complexion, leaving it soft and radiant. It is also effectively used in remedies to clear our skin of blackheads, pimples, acne, and blemishes. Furthermore, it is employed with other ingredients to hamper the growth of unwanted facial hair, fix any instances of uneven pigmentation, and reduce the appearance of dark circles *and* lines on our neck. Used on hair, gram flour aids in fighting dandruff, strengthening brittle hair, and restoring the shine in dull or dry hair.

Grapes (Green) or Grape Juice

Green grapes contain silica, a vital mineral used by our bodies to maintain the healthy growth of skin, hair, and nails. This affords them their ability to repair and revive our skin cells—they are therefore effective when used in remedies to treat dry skin, further minimizing the occurrence of fine lines and wrinkles. In addition, the acid contained in grape juice qualifies it as a gentle, but effective, astringent; its use is known to aid in clearing troubled skin of pimples, acne, and blemishes.

Henna

Used on our hair, henna performs two simultaneous functions—it colors, *and* it conditions. As a natural source of color, henna imparts a rich, brownish-red color to black or brunette hair. As a conditioner, henna revives dull or dry hair *or* softens normal hair by sealing each cuticle, thus locking in our natural oils. This very ability to condition allows henna to promote a healthy scalp, not only reducing hair loss, but, on the contrary, inducing hair growth. (Note: Always use *only* natural henna on your hair; commercially produced henna that comes in a range of colors contains chemicals and dyes that may harm your skin and hair.)

Honey

Well-known by our ancestors for its nourishing benefits, honey has been used as a natural beauty aid for centuries. It contains silica, a vital mineral used by our bodies to maintain the healthy growth of skin, hair, and nails. It is therefore very effective when used in remedies to treat dark circles, as well as brittle nails. Like glycerin, honey is a humectant as well—it attracts moisture to our skin, and then helps our skin to retain that moisture, helping us attain a supple and radiant complexion. This attribute also enables it to successfully treat dry skin, further preventing or reducing the occurrence of fine lines and wrinkles. In addition, honey possesses antibacterial properties that promote the healing of pimples,

acne, scars, and blemishes. All in all, due to each one of its restorative properties, this ingredient validates its use in *just about any* remedy.

Lemon

Loaded with Vitamin C, the ever-versatile lemon is highly regarded for its ability to be used in a multitude of remedies for both our skin and hair. Due to its high content of natural acid, its juice effectively dissolves any excess deposits on the surface of our skin and hair, qualifying it as a potent, antiseptic astringent—it is especially effective when used on oily skin to restore its moisture balance—it cleans out any clogged pores, therefore making an excellent remedy for blackheads, pimples, and acne. As a natural bleaching agent for our skin, lemon juice lightens our complexion, as well as reduces the appearance of blemishes, freckles, and dark circles, *and* the occurrence of uneven pigmentation; it can also be used on our nails to reduce any discoloration. Used on hair, this fruit has proven itself effective in treating dandruff and oily hair, as well as restoring the luster to dull or dry hair by cleansing it of any shampoo or styling product build-up. It is further known to successfully prevent any occurrences of hair loss and premature graying because of its ability to cleanse out any blocked pores on our scalp, thereby enabling a better absorption of vital nutrients by our hair roots. This very ability also allows lemon juice to promote a more rapid healing when used on our skin to treat fine lines and wrinkles, dry skin, and hardened or cracked skin on the soles of our feet.

ABOUT THE INGREDIENTS

Lentils (Green)

Green lentils are loaded with protein. A coarsely ground, green lentil facemask provides immense nourishment to our skin, while its texture qualifies it as an excellent exfoliating scrub.

Milk

Milk is one of the most inexpensive anti-wrinkle treatments that money can buy! It contains lactic acid, which is a pure indulgence for dry or depleted skin—this nourishing quality allows it to be effectively used in remedies to not only attain a smooth and radiant complexion, but also prevent fine lines and wrinkles. Milk is very cooling and soothing for our skin, and is therefore also used in a multitude of remedies to soothe tired and puffy eyes, treat sunburn, as well as cure pimples and acne. Used with other ingredients, milk is further known to lighten our complexion, fix any occurrences of uneven pigmentation, and reduce the appearance of dark circles and blemishes. It makes an effective cleanser, without robbing our skin of its natural oils.

Mint Leaves (Fresh)

Primarily known for its culinary uses, mint is, however, also very commonly found as an ingredient in a wide variety of skincare products that promote themselves to be "cooling" for our skin. Mint leaves possess antibacterial

properties that qualify them as a mild antiseptic; used in remedies with other ingredients, they lend our skin a healthy glow, as well as reduce, if not eliminate, pimples, acne, blemishes, dark circles, and instances of uneven pigmentation. Their juice makes an effective cleanser and toner for our skin, (*including* that on our scalp)—its use is therefore also known to successfully combat oily hair.

Mustard Oil

Mustard oil is potent and has a heating effect; when used on our skin (*including* that on our scalp), it not only infuses moisture, but also stimulates the circulation of blood—it is therefore very effective for treating both dandruff and hair loss. Additionally, it possesses antibacterial properties that enable it to aid in curing any cracks or fissures that form on the soles of our feet.

Neem Oil or Powder

Neem oil makes an excellent remedy for hair and scalp-related problems—its use not only infuses shine, but also strengthens our hair roots and strands by infusing moisture, allowing it to successfully aid in fighting occurrences of dandruff and hair loss. Used in either form, neem is also highly effective in replenishing the moisture in our skin—it not only leaves it feeling soft and supple, but also lends it a healthy glow. This ingredient further possesses cooling properties and is used as an aid in remedies to clear troubled skin of pimples and their accompanying blemishes.

Olive Oil

Olive oil is rich in vitamins and antioxidants. It is used in remedies for both our skin and hair. Used on skin, it demonstrates its ability to heal by soothing and repairing dry, sore, or inflamed skin—it is *just as* effective on the delicate skin around our eyes, as it is on the tough skin on the soles of our feet. Olive oil is further known for its ability to revitalize a dull complexion; it does so by infusing the skin with immense moisture. This *very* attribute also allows it to demonstrate its effectiveness when used to treat hair and scalp-related problems, such as dandruff, dry hair, and hair loss. Additionally, this ingredient treats brittle nails by nourishing them, thereby restoring their strength.

Oranges or Orange Juice

Oranges are abundant in their content of natural acid. Their juice therefore makes an excellent astringent—it cleanses out our pores by extracting any excess dirt and oil from them and is effectively used on oily skin to restore its moisture balance; this further prevents the occurrence of blackheads, pimples, and acne. This fruit contains a liberal amount of Vitamin C and antioxidants that prevent and cure skin damage; it has therefore also found use in remedies to repair dry skin and help it attain a luxurious glow, as well as reduce the appearance of fine lines, wrinkles, and blemishes.

ABOUT THE INGREDIENTS

Papaya

The use of papaya in skincare remedies has proven to be both preventative and restorative. Especially rich in enzymes that dissolve any dead cells on the surface of our skin, this fruit is very effective when used as a cleanser. If you think that its seeds serve no purpose, think again! Crushed papaya seeds not only make an *excellent* exfoliant, but are also known to possess properties that help minimize the fine lines and wrinkles caused by sun damage. Furthermore, the papaya is rich in vitamins that nourish and replenish our skin, leaving it feeling soft and supple. It is also used in a wide variety of remedies to lend radiance to a dull complexion, balance oily skin, and reduce the appearance of uneven pigmentation. (Note: Due to its rich content of enzymes, make sure that you limit the use of any mask that contains either papaya or its juice to *no more than* 5–10 minutes.)

Pineapples or Pineapple Juice

Rich in vitamins, minerals, and enzymes, pineapples make an excellent skin softener. Their use revitalizes dull and dry skin, especially that on coarse areas, such as our knees, elbows, and heels. Pineapple juice is high in acid content; it is therefore effective when used as an astringent on our skin to dissolve dirt, oil, and bacteria—it is ideal for skin that is troubled by pimples and acne. Furthermore, the rich acid content in pineapple juice also stimulates our skin brilliantly, making it effective when used in remedies to treat fine lines and wrinkles.

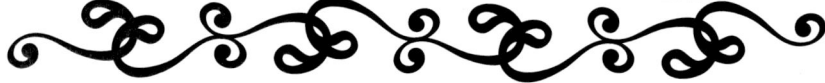

ABOUT THE INGREDIENTS

Potatoes

Potatoes contain a number of important vitamins and minerals. Used externally, they help restore the moisture balance in oily skin, thus preventing the subsequent occurrence of pimples and acne. They are also effective when used in remedies to lighten a dark or dull complexion *and* reduce the appearance of scars or blemishes, freckles, and dark circles. Furthermore, the starch contained in them possesses anti-inflammatory properties, which allows them to aid in reducing the puffiness around our eyes. Like carrots and cucumbers, the benefits of potatoes lie in their skin—they are the most effective when used unpeeled.

Rosewater

Distilled from rose petals, this floral water possesses mild astringent properties—so mild, in fact, that it has instead found use as a gentle, but amazingly restorative, toner. It also possesses the tremendous ability to cool and soothe. Furthermore, as its name suggests, *rosewater* is the gateway to petal-soft skin. With all these attributes combined, rosewater validates its use in *just about any* remedy for our skin. (Note: Use only the 100% pure form of rosewater, which does not contain any preservatives. Also, if possible, store your rosewater in the refrigerator—used cold on our skin, it is extra-refreshing. If you have an ice-cube tray at home, make ice-cubes using this floral water; use these in place of your over-the-counter toner.)

ABOUT THE INGREDIENTS

Salt (Table)

Over and above being a critical ingredient in our food, salt has proven its usefulness even when used externally on both our skin and hair. It possesses powerful antibacterial properties and has been recognized for its ability to heal by drawing out impurities from our skin. A water-soak with salt helps soothe tired feet, as well as soften and disinfect hardened soles. Furthermore, salt is used in remedies to reduce the bags or any puffiness under our eyes. Due to its texture, it also makes an effective exfoliant for our skin. Used with other ingredients on hair, salt aids in reducing the occurrence of dandruff.

Sandalwood Powder

Known for its sensual, woody aroma, sandalwood powder is a proven healer of stubbornly oily skin. This, in turn, allows it to prevent the formation of blackheads, pimples, acne, and blemishes. Like rosewater, sandalwood powder possesses tremendous cooling properties, to the extent that it makes a very effective, natural substitute for over-the-counter foot powders that are available for foot perspiration. Furthermore, used on dry or cracked skin on the soles of our feet, this ingredient relieves itching and inflammation. It is also known for its remarkable ability to tone and condition our skin; its use in remedies helps us attain soft and supple skin.

Sesame Oil or Seeds

Abundant in vitamins and minerals, sesame has been used for thousands of years by people around the world. It is primarily known for its culinary uses; however, it has also been found to demonstrate extraordinary healing powers when used externally. Used in either form, this ingredient possesses antioxidant properties that aid in slowing down the process of aging. In analyzing beneficial oils for skincare, sesame oil ranks high among other popular oils such as Vitamin E, coconut, and almond, because of its unique ability to be easily absorbed by our skin, thereby immensely nourishing it *and* stimulating and detoxifying even its deepest layers. Its use has therefore also been known to effectively combat dry skin, revive a dull complexion, treat pimples and acne, and fade the appearance of blemishes, dark circles and instances of uneven pigmentation.

Strawberries

Strawberries are rich in salicylic acid, an ingredient found in many commercial acne creams. They therefore make a *very* effective remedy for skin that is troubled by pimples and acne. Mashed to a pulp, this fruit makes an excellent exfoliant for our skin, leaving it refreshed, conditioned, *and* toned.

ABOUT THE INGREDIENTS

Sugar

Like glycerin and honey, sugar is a humectant as well—it attracts moisture to our skin, and then helps our skin to retain that moisture. Due to its coarse texture, it is very effective as an exfoliant—a scrub made using sugar granules both soothes and moisturizes as it sloughs off any dead cells on the surface of our skin.

Tomatoes or Tomato Juice

Tomatoes contain one of nature's most powerful antioxidants, lycopene, which possesses the ability to be easily absorbed by our skin. They are further abundant in natural acids, which allows their juice to act as an excellent astringent—it cleanses out our pores by extracting any excess dirt and oil from them, and is especially effective when used on oily skin to restore its moisture balance. Their rich acid content also stimulates our skin brilliantly, allowing tomato juice to effectively treat fine lines and wrinkles. Furthermore, tomatoes act as a great toner as well—they refine our pores and refresh our skin. They are effectively used in remedies to reduce the appearance of freckles or dark circles, lighten a dark or dull complexion, and help our skin attain a radiant glow.

Turmeric Powder

Primarily known for its culinary uses, turmeric powder is also referred to as a *Miracle Spice* due to its tremendous healing power when used externally. It possesses powerful antibacterial and anti-inflammatory properties, and also contains curcumin, a compound that is considered to be a potent antioxidant. It is successfully used to treat split or fissured skin on the soles of our feet. Furthermore, over the centuries, due to its versatility, turmeric powder has been used with other ingredients in a multitude of remedies to cure pimples and acne, restore the radiance in a dark or dull complexion, reduce the appearance of blemishes or dark circles *and* any instances of uneven pigmentation, and reduce, if not eliminate, unwanted facial hair. All in all, this spice has earned an undisputable reputation for its ability to cure a vast range of imperfections in our skin.

Vinegar

Due to its high acid content, vinegar is known for its ability to effectively dissolve any excess deposits on the surface of both our skin and hair. Used on skin, it reduces scaling and peeling, (*including* that on our scalp)—it is therefore effective in remedies to treat the occurrence of dandruff. Used on hair, it further aids in neutralizing oily hair and cleansing our strands of any build-up caused by shampoo and styling products, thereby exposing their natural sheen. Vinegar also acts as a stimulant when applied, promoting the circulation of blood; it is effective when used on our skin to relieve the stinging sensation caused by sunburn. (Note: In employing this ingredient in any remedy, make sure that you use a high-quality apple cider vinegar. Also, when using it in any hair-related remedies, bear in mind that vinegar adds highlights to brunette hair.)

Vitamin E Oil

Vitamin E is an antioxidant that binds environmental toxins in our skin and promotes cell respiration; it is therefore recognized for its ability to prevent or reduce the appearance of dark circles and age spots. Vitamin E oil possesses anti-inflammatory properties; used on skin, it not only soothes, but also moisturizes, leaving our skin feeling soft and supple. It is especially effective when used to treat the occurrence of fine lines and wrinkles, as well as dry or sun-damaged skin, but is also used to reduce the puffiness around eyes. (Note: When employing this ingredient in your remedies, you can either use separately-bought Vitamin E oil *or* Vitamin E capsules—any potency is okay. If you choose to use the latter, simply prick or cut open a capsule and squeeze out its contents.)

Watermelon

Watermelon contains concentrated amounts of one of nature's most powerful antioxidants, lycopene, which possesses the ability to be easily absorbed by

our skin. This fruit also possesses mild astringent properties. Combined, these attributes allow watermelon juice to act as an excellent cleanser when used in remedies to treat clogged pores and blackheads, as well as pimples, acne, and blemishes. Additionally, due to its high water content, watermelon is tremendously cooling for our skin, which allows its juice to act as an effective skin toner as well. This fruit further contains vitamins that enable it to nourish and condition our skin, leaving it feeling soft and supple.

Whole Wheat Flour

Whole wheat flour is rich in its content of fiber; this, in turn, contributes to its texture, allowing it to act as an effective exfoliant. Used with other ingredients, it aids in the removal of unwanted facial hair. This ingredient also contains Vitamin E; its use, therefore, has a rejuvenating effect on our skin.

Yogurt (Plain)

Rich in its content of vitamins and minerals, yogurt is extremely versatile as a beauty aid—it is used in a multitude of remedies for both our skin and hair. It possesses tremendous cooling properties; its use on skin shrinks large pores, thereby discouraging any dirt and oil from depositing in them—this, in turn, prevents the formation of blackheads. It is abundant in lactic acid, and therefore also aids in reducing the appearance of dark circles and blemishes, *as well as* any instances of uneven pigmentation. Yogurt possesses

ABOUT THE INGREDIENTS

antibacterial properties, which further allows its use on our skin to aid in healing occurrences of pimples and acne. Used on hair in combination with other ingredients, it is known to cure dandruff, strengthen brittle hair, and prevent premature graying *and* hair loss. Its use infuses moisture in dry or dull hair *and* skin, leaving both feeling nourished. (Note: When using this ingredient in any remedy, *always* use plain yogurt. Also, when using it in any hair-related remedies, allow it to warm to room temperature before you apply it—applying cold yogurt could cause a headache.)

WHERE YOU CAN FIND THE INGREDIENTS

Most of the ingredients referenced in this book (such as honey, olive oil, fruits, vegetables, dairy products, etc.) are *very* commonly available at your local grocery store; you can conveniently find the ones that are not, at *any* Indian store—visit www.Indi-Yeah.com to search for Indian grocers in your area.